LOW SODIUM COOKING
from the
HEART

Happy Cooking Mel!

Pam

PAMELA VIVIAN

MERRY XMAS
RICHARD + ROSA

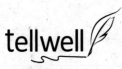

Tellwell Talent
www.tellwell.ca

ISBN
978-0-2288-3440-3 (Hardcover)
978-0-2288-3439-7 (Paperback)
978-0-2288-3441-0 (eBook)

This book is dedicated to my wonderful husband, children, grandchildren, family and many friends who all make my life worth living. It comes from my heart and I hope the contents are enjoyed by many.

Photography by Tara Stolar

Edited by Allison Ashton

Prologue

It is quite shocking to be given the news that you have hepatitis C and cirrhosis of the liver. Yes, you know you have not been feeling up to snuff lately: tired, lethargic, not sleeping well and your stomach has been a little off but nothing you feel you should really go and bother your doctor about. Doesn't everyone go through these stages once in a while?

Then all of a sudden your belly swells and there is a war going on in there and off to Emergency you go. Next comes the diagnosis of hepatitis C and cirrhosis.

After that, all chaos breaks out in your body. For those that also suffer with this and are wondering what symptoms other people have, the following are some of mine:

Inability to think

Pain in muscles, joints and bones

Dizziness and poor balance

Reduced vision

Hair loss

Terrible skin and nails

Itchy skin and stinging red spots

Muscle cramps and twitching

Restless legs

Shaky

Weight loss

Not sleeping

Extreme tiredness

No energy

Cold

Inflammation especially in pelvic area at night

Upset and very noisy stomach (Oh the agony sometimes, sharp pains, dull ache, etc.)

Nausea and vomiting

Fluid retention and swelling

Memory loss - forget people, places and things

The whole world revolving when you lay flat in bed - holding on so you don't fall off

All of these symptoms come and go from hour to hour and day to day. At one point I could barely walk, talk or see. Thinking was impossible. This made planning an outing difficult especially with the washroom issues. Now that the hepatitis C has been treated the symptoms are not as bad as they were but still considerable.

Quite frequently I will be working in the kitchen or garden and a veil of weariness descends over me and I need to go and rest for 10 or 15 minutes.

After 4 o'clock in the afternoon the symptoms seem to be worse. Apparently, this is because your brain is tired and cannot deal with all of this anymore for the day.

The other big issue of living with liver disease is that the treatment is laxatives and diuretics. So we live in the washroom. When you do go out, you make sure you know where the washroom is anywhere you go because your life revolves around it. Then there is the flatulence from the laxatives that can be very embarrassing.

I do hope this helps some fellow sufferers and, also, others to understand a little of what it is like to live with this disease. Facing death makes you appreciate every minute you have. Today my days revolve around medications and the effects of them but no matter how much discomfort or pain there is I am grateful every day for being here to enjoy spending time with the ones I love. The best thing you can do is just keep on smiling and live your life to the fullest possible.

One thing that also changes is your diet. Low sodium it is and from that came this book.

Cooking Tips

In the summer, cooking low sodium is fairly simple, put some meat on the barbeque with a salad or vegetables as side dishes. In the winter it is more difficult. Hopefully, these tips and recipes will make it a little easier.

Use grated Parmesan cheese from the deli. It is more expensive but is much lower in sodium; however, some varieties are lower than others.

Read labels. There is one tomato paste that has 1% sodium. You will find other products with reduced sodium amounts too. I have been unable to locate low sodium cheese to try it. If low sodium cans are not available rinsing contents with water to reduce sodium will help depending on the contents (e.g. beans, corn etc.). When choosing low sodium products read nutritional facts tables. Any products <5% is a little and anything >15% is a lot.

Let beef come to room temperature before cooking.

Coat steaks with a layer of oil so spices will stick. Kirkland (Costco brand) has an organic no-salt seasoning with 1% sodium. This is an excellent steak spice.

Use fresh chocolate for melting for a smoother nicer melted chocolate.

Use fresh ingredients (fruit, vegetables and herbs) whenever possible. There is a big difference in the taste.

Use fresh breadcrumbs as well so you can control the salt content better and they taste better.

The ration for fresh versus dried herbs and spices is three fresh for one dried. (three fresh teaspoons versus one dried of parsley or any other).

Use spices and fruits to make meats tastier without using salt. Beef is the most difficult because it loves being paired with salt. Other low sodium sauces make meat tasty too.

The nutritional facts are guides only and percentages will vary depending on the content of brands purchased. Look for low sodium cheeses. I was unable to find any in my area but you may have better luck.

Choosing well trimmed meats, skinless meats, limiting added sugars and eating well balanced meals (including proteins, vegetables, fruits and whole grains) will lead to a healthier lifestyle.

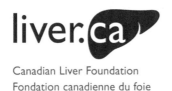

Canadian Liver Foundation
Fondation canadienne du foie

Bringing liver research to life
Donner vie à la recherche sur le foie

Weighing in at a little over one kilogram, your liver is a complex chemical factory that works 24 hours a day. It processes virtually everything you eat, drink, breathe in or rub on your skin; in fact, the liver performs more than 500 functions that are vital to life. Every day, your liver helps your body by providing it with energy, fighting off infections and toxins, helping clot the blood, regulating hormones and much, much more.

1 in 4 Canadians may be affected by liver disease, including everyone from newborns to older adults. The liver is a resilient organ that is easy to ignore – until something goes wrong. Because of its wide-ranging responsibilities, your healthy liver can come under attack by viruses, toxic substances, contaminants and diseases. However, even when under siege, the liver is very slow to complain. People who have problems with their liver are frequently unaware because they may have few, if any, symptoms. Your liver is such a determined organ that it will continue working even when two-thirds of it has been damaged.

Cirrhosis is a condition (not a disease) that can happen when any form of liver disease reaches an advanced stage where there is permanent damage or scarring of the liver. This leads to a blockage of blood flow through the liver and prevents normal metabolic and regulatory processes.

The body needs some sodium to function, however, for those who are living with cirrhosis and have decreased liver function, a balanced, low-sodium, low-sugar diet is an important part of a liver-healthy lifestyle. Too much sodium can worsen the symptoms of cirrhosis, so people who have advanced liver disease and cirrhosis should consume less than 2,000 mg of sodium per day. Following a low-sodium diet is not as simple as getting rid of the saltshaker. In addition to not adding salt to food, it is important to cook and eat foods with low-sodium contents.

The Canadian Liver Foundation recognizes the importance of healthful living as prevention, management and treatment for many liver diseases and conditions, including for those who are living with cirrhosis.

For more information on liver health, visit www.liver.ca.

3100 Steeles Avenue East, Suite 801, Markham, ON L3R 8T3 • 416 491-3353 • Toll Free: 1 800 563-5483 • Fax: 905 752-1540
Canadian Charitable Registration No. 10686 2949 RR0001

Table of Contents

Vinegars, Dressings and Sauces

Tarragon Vinegar..2

Bearnaise Sauce..3

Strawberry Vinaigrette..4

Lime Ginger Mayo...5

Salads and Soups

Broccoli Salad...8

Citrus Salad..9

Strawberry Spinach Salad...10

Honey and Orange Salad..11

Egg Salad...12

Layered Fruit Salad..13

Carrot-Raisin Salad...14

Chilled Strawberry Soup...15

Cheese and Broccoli Soup..16

Cauliflower Soup..17

Beef

Beef Enchiladas..20

Beef Tips in Slow Cooker...21

Beef Roll Ups...22

Beef Stroganoff..23

Porcupine Meatballs...24

Salisbury Steak...25

Ground Beef Dinner...26

Macaroni Meat...27

Chicken

Chicken Alfredo 30

Chicken Enchiladas 31

Chicken/Turkey Pot Pie 32

Grilled Chicken with Lemon Asparagus Pasta 33

Saucy French Onion Chicken 34

Tomato Basil Chicken 35

Miscellaneous

Macaroni and Cheese 38

Manicotti 39

Moon Chilli 40

Pancake Batter 41

Pasta Sauce 42

Potatoes Romanoff 43

Scalloped Potatoes 44

Sunshine Jam 45

Pork

Pork Chops 48

Pork Chops and Rice 49

Spiced Apple Pork Roast 50

Apricot Pork Roast 51

Vegetables

Asparagus with Zesty Hollandaise Sauce 54

Broccoli Casserole 55

Beets 56

Caramelized Ginger Carrots 57

Green Beans 58

Carrots and Asparagus 59

Stuffed Green Peppers 60

Vegetable Fettuccine 61

Vegetable Casserole 62

Desserts

Cranberry Pineapple Frozen Dessert 64

Exquisite Lemon Pie 65

Crème Caramel 66

Sparkling Raspberry Pie 67

Banana Coconut Cream Pie 68

Berry Custard Dessert 69

Thanksgiving Cheesecake 71

Creamy Chocolate Dessert 72

Lemon Pudding Cups 73

Icy Dark Sweet Cherries 74

Orange Chiffon Pie 75

Fresh Strawberry Pie 76

Chocolate Cake 77

Chocolate Brownie Cake 78

Carrot Cake 79

White Cake 81

Banana Cake 82

VINEGARS, DRESSINGS AND SAUCES

1. Tarragon Vinegar

2. Bearnaise Sauce

3. Strawberry Vinaigrette

4. Lime Ginger Mayo

Tarragon Vinegar

I have been unable to find this so I make my own from a recipe given to me by my friend Georgie.

Serves 16

4 sprigs of fresh tarragon
1 peeled garlic clove
2 (1 inch) squares lemon peel
5 black pepper corns
White vinegar

Put all ingredients into a 1-pint jar or decorative jar. Fill with vinegar. Let stand for 4 weeks. Will keep up to a year.

Tarragon Vinegar

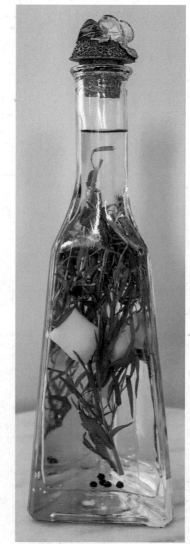

Nutrition Facts

16 servings per container

Serving size	**(28g)**

Amount Per Serving

Calories	**5**

	% Daily Value*
Total Fat 0g	0%
Saturated Fat 0g	0%
Trans Fat 0g	
Cholesterol 0mg	0%
Sodium 0mg	0%
Total Carbohydrate 2g	1%
Dietary Fiber <1g	2%
Total Sugars 0g	
Includes 0g Added Sugars	0%
Protein 0g	
Vitamin D 0mcg	0%
Calcium 10mg	0%
Iron 0.2mg	0%
Potassium 0mg	0%

* The % Daily Value (DV) tells you how much a nutrient in a serving of food contributes to a daily diet. 2,000 calories a day is used for general nutrition advice.

INGREDIENTS: DISTILLED VINEGAR, BLACK PEPPER, TARRAGON, LEMON PEEL, GARLIC

Tarragon Vinegar

Bearnaise Sauce

Serves 12

This is a family favourite at our house, awesome in place of gravy for beef. Bearnaise sauce is believed to be created by Chef Collinet in 1836 for the opening of Le Pavillion Henri IV, a restaurant just outside of Paris. King Henry IV was believed to be a gourmet cook and came from the region of Bearn. We tried the recipe using both salted and unsalted butter. Everyone seemed to like it both ways. It was a little sweeter tasting using unsalted butter.

3/4 cup white wine (alcoholic or non-alcoholic)
2 Tbsp tarragon vinegar
2 Tbsp finely chopped onion
1/2 tsp dried tarragon
1 tsp dried parsley
2 crushed peppercorns
3 egg yolks
1/2 cup melted butter (salted, unsalted or half salted and half unsalted)
(I have done the nutrition guide with salted butter)

Combine wine, onion, tarragon, parsley and peppercorns in a small saucepan. Boil until reduced to one third of original quantity. Let cool. Melt butter and let cool. Add egg yolks to cooled vinegar combination and add butter. Whisk together over heat stirring continuously until the sauce has the consistency of whipped cream. If the sauce should curdle, whisk in a teaspoon or two of cold water.

Nutritional label is done using salted butter. Sodium content would be less using half salted and half unsalted.

Bernaise Sauce

Nutrition Facts

12 servings per container

Serving size	(25g)

Amount Per Serving	
Calories	**90**

	% Daily Value*
Total Fat 9g	12%
Saturated Fat 5g	25%
Trans Fat 0g	
Cholesterol 60mg	20%
Sodium 65mg	3%
Total Carbohydrate <1g	0%
Dietary Fiber 0g	0%
Total Sugars 0g	
Includes 0g Added Sugars	0%
Protein 1g	

Vitamin D 0.2mcg	0%
Calcium 10mg	0%
Iron 0.2mg	0%
Potassium 20mg	0%

* The % Daily Value (DV) tells you how much a nutrient in a serving of food contributes to a daily diet. 2,000 calories a day is used for general nutrition advice.

INGREDIENTS: WHITE WINE, BUTTER (CREAM, SALT), TARRAGON VINEGAR, EGG YOLK, ONIONS, BLACK PEPPER, PARSLEY, TARRAGON

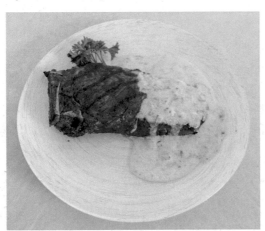

Bearnaise sauce

3

Strawberry Vinaigrette

Serves 2

Other fruits could be used to change up the menu.

1 Tbsp apple cider vinegar

1 Tbsp lemon juice

Sugar to taste if desired

2 medium strawberries

Combine all ingredients in a blender or food processor. Puree until smooth. Pour over salad.

Strawberry Vinaigrette

Nutrition Facts

Serving Size: (29g)
Servings Per Container: 2

Amount Per Serving

Calories 10 | Calories from Fat 0

% Daily Value*

Total Fat 0g	**0%**
Saturated Fat 0g	**0%**
Trans Fat 0g	
Cholesterol 0mg	**0%**
Sodium 0mg	**0%**
Total Carbohydrate 2g	**1%**
Dietary Fiber 0g	**0%**
Sugars 1g	
Protein 0g	

Vitamin A 0%	•	Vitamin C 15%
Calcium 0%	•	Iron 0%

* Percent Daily Values are based on a 2,000 calorie diet. Your daily values may be higher or lower depending on your calorie needs:

	Calories:	2,000	2,500
Total Fat	Less than	65g	80g
Sat Fat	Less than	20g	25g
Cholesterol	Less than	300mg	300mg
Sodium	Less than	2,400mg	2,400mg
Total Carbohydrate		300g	375g
Dietary Fiber		25g	30g

INGREDIENTS: STRAWBERRIES, LEMON JUICE, APPLE CIDER VINEGAR, SUGAR

Lime Ginger Mayo

This sauce is excellent served with fish or chicken.

1/2 cup Miracle Whip™

1/8 cup plain yogurt

1/2 tsp finely grated fresh ginger

1 tsp finely grated lime rind

2 tsp lime juice

Mix all ingredients in a bowl and serve.

Lime Ginger Mayo

Nutrition Facts	
12 servings per container	
Serving size	**(15g)**

Amount Per Serving	
Calories	**25**

	% Daily Value*
Total Fat 2g	**3%**
Saturated Fat 0g	**0%**
Trans Fat 1.5g	
Cholesterol <5mg	**1%**
Sodium 80mg	**3%**
Total Carbohydrate 2g	**1%**
Dietary Fiber 0g	**0%**
Total Sugars 1g	
Includes 0g Added Sugars	**0%**
Protein 1g	
Vitamin D 0mcg	0%
Calcium 10mg	0%
Iron 0mg	0%
Potassium 10mg	0%

* The % Daily Value (DV) tells you how much a nutrient in a serving of food contributes to a daily diet. 2,000 calories a day is used for general nutrition advice.

INGREDIENTS: SALAD DRESSING, KRAFT MIRACLE WHIP LIGHT DRESSING, NONFAT GREEK YOGURT (NONFAT YOGURT (CULTURED PASTEURIZED NONFAT MILK), LIVE AND ACTIVE CULTURES: S. THERMOPHILUS, L. BULGARICUS, L. ACIDOPHILUS, BIFIDUS AND L. CASEI), LIME JUICE, LIME ZEST, GINGER

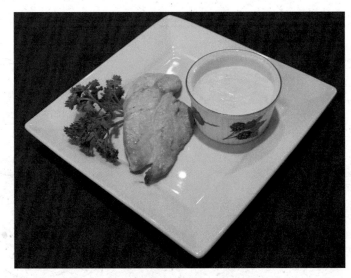

Lime Ginger Mayo

SALADS AND SOUPS

1. Broccoli Salad

2. Citrus Salad

3. Strawberry Spinach Salad

4. Honey and Orange Salad

5. Egg Salad

6. Layered Fruit Salad

7. Carrot-Raisin Salad

8. Chilled Strawberry Soup

9. Cheese and Broccoli Soup

10. Cauliflower Soup

Broccoli Salad

This recipe can be made many different ways using various nut and dried fruit combinations.

Serves 6-8 as a side dish

3 cups broccoli florets
1/4 cup chopped red onion
1/4 cup salt-free nuts (chopped pecans, chopped peanuts, sunflower seeds, etc.)
1/4 cup dried fruit (raisins, dried cranberries, dried currants, etc.)

Dressing

1/2 cup Miracle Whip™
1/8 cup white sugar
1/2 Tbsp red wine vinegar

Mix dressing well and pour over broccoli, nuts and fruit. Toss to coat. Chill.

Broccoli Salad

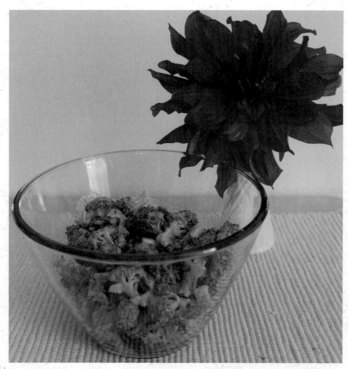

Broccoli Salad

Nutrition Facts

6 servings per container

Serving size	(92g)

Amount Per Serving

Calories 130

	% Daily Value*
Total Fat 7g	9%
Saturated Fat 1g	5%
Trans Fat 3g	
Cholesterol <5mg	2%
Sodium 170mg	7%
Total Carbohydrate 17g	6%
Dietary Fiber 2g	7%
Total Sugars 12g	
Includes 5g Added Sugars	10%
Protein 2g	
Vitamin D 0mcg	0%
Calcium 30mg	2%
Iron 0.7mg	4%
Potassium 240mg	6%

* The % Daily Value (DV) tells you how much a nutrient in a serving of food contributes to a daily diet. 2,000 calories a day is used for general nutrition advice.

INGREDIENTS: BROCCOLI, SALAD DRESSING, KRAFT MIRACLE WHIP LIGHT DRESSING, RED ONION, RAISINS, SUGAR, PECANS, RED WINE VINEGAR

Citrus Salad

Serves 4

Dressing Ingredients

2 Tbsp vegetable oil
2 Tbsp apple cider vinegar
2 Tbsp honey

Salad Ingredients

4 cups torn leaf lettuce
1/4 cup chopped red onion
1/4 cup fresh parsley
2 oranges, pared, sectioned and drained
2 grapefruit, pared, sectioned and drained

Pared means peeling including the outer membrane. Sectioned means cutting between slices, removing the membrane.

Combine salad ingredients in a large serving bowl. In a small bowl mix honey, vinegar and oil and stir. Pour over salad and toss to coat.

Citrus Salad

Nutrition Facts	
4 servings per container	
Serving size	**(191g)**
Amount Per Serving	
Calories	**160**
	% Daily Value*
Total Fat 7g	**9%**
Saturated Fat 0.5g	**3%**
Trans Fat 0g	
Cholesterol 0mg	**0%**
Sodium 20mg	**1%**
Total Carbohydrate 23g	**8%**
Dietary Fiber 3g	**11%**
Total Sugars 18g	
Includes 9g Added Sugars	**18%**
Protein 2g	
Vitamin D 0mcg	0%
Calcium 70mg	6%
Iron 1.4mg	8%
Potassium 320mg	6%

* The % Daily Value (DV) tells you how much a nutrient in a serving of food contributes to a daily diet. 2,000 calories a day is used for general nutrition advice.

INGREDIENTS: GRAPEFRUIT, RAW, PINK AND RED, ALL AREAS, ORANGES, LETTUCE, PARSLEY, RED ONION, HONEY, APPLE CIDER VINEGAR, OIL, VEGETABLE, NATREON CANOLA, HIGH STABILITY, NON TRANS, HIGH OLEIC (70%)

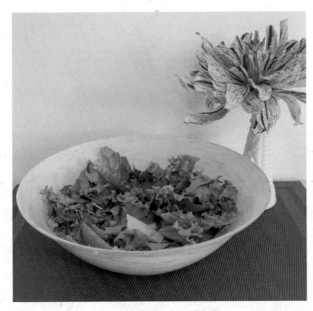

Citrus Salad

Strawberry Spinach Salad

Dressing Ingredients

2 Tbsp sesame seeds

1 Tbsp poppy seeds

1/2 cup white sugar

1/2 cup olive oil

1/4 cup white vinegar

1/4 tsp paprika

1/4 tsp Worcestershire sauce

1 Tbsp finely minced onion

Salad Ingredients

10 oz fresh baby spinach

1 quart sliced strawberries

1/4 cup slivered almonds

In a medium bowl, whisk together all dressing ingredients. Cover and chill one hour.

In a large bowl, combine salad ingredients. Pour dressing over salad and toss. Refrigerate for 10-15 minutes before serving.

Strawberry Spinach Salad

Nutrition Facts

10 servings per container

Serving size	(325g)

Amount Per Serving

Calories	240

	% Daily Value*
Total Fat 14g	**18%**
Saturated Fat 2g	**10%**
Trans Fat 0g	
Cholesterol 0mg	**0%**
Sodium 170mg	**7%**
Total Carbohydrate 25g	**9%**
Dietary Fiber 7g	**25%**
Total Sugars 15g	
Includes 11g Added Sugars	**22%**
Protein 7g	
Vitamin D 0mcg	0%
Calcium 240mg	20%
Iron 7.4mg	40%
Potassium 140mg	2%

* The % Daily Value (DV) tells you how much a nutrient in a serving of food contributes to a daily diet. 2,000 calories a day is used for general nutrition advice.

INGREDIENTS: SPINACH, STRAWBERRIES, SUGAR, OLIVE OIL, DISTILLED VINEGAR, ALMONDS, ONIONS, SESAME SEEDS, POPPY SEEDS, WORCESTERSHIRE SAUCE (DISTILLED WHITE VINEGAR, ANCHOVIES, GARLIC, MOLASSES, ONIONS, SALT, SUGAR, WATER, CHILI PEPPER EXTRACT, CLOVES, NATURAL FLAVORINGS, TAMARIND EXTRACT), PAPRIKA

Honey and Orange Salad

Six lunch servings

Dressing Ingredients

1/4 cup sugar

8 tsp lemon juice

2 Tbsp vinegar

5 tsp honey

1/2 tsp ground mustard

1/2 tsp paprika

1/8 tsp celery seed

1/2 cup vegetable oil

leaf lettuce

6 oranges pared and sliced (peeled including membrane)

In a blender or food processor combine sugar, lemon juice, vinegar, honey, mustard, paprika, celery seed and vegetable oil. Blend until slightly thickened. Pour into a jar and chill. Line plates with a bed of lettuce and arrange orange slices on top. Shake dressing and drizzle over oranges.

Honey and Orange Salad

Nutrition Facts	
6 servings per container	
Serving size	**(235g)**

Amount Per Serving	
Calories	**300**

	% Daily Value*
Total Fat 19g	**24%**
Saturated Fat 1.5g	**8%**
Trans Fat 0g	
Cholesterol 0mg	**0%**
Sodium 15mg	**1%**
Total Carbohydrate 33g	**12%**
Dietary Fiber 4g	**14%**
Total Sugars 28g	
Includes 14g Added Sugars	**28%**
Protein 2g	
Vitamin D 0mcg	0%
Calcium 80mg	6%
Iron 0.7mg	4%
Potassium 350mg	8%

* The % Daily Value (DV) tells you how much a nutrient in a serving of food contributes to a daily diet. 2,000 calories a day is used for general nutrition advice.

INGREDIENTS: ORANGES, LETTUCE, OIL, VEGETABLE, NATREON CANOLA, HIGH STABILITY, NON TRANS, HIGH OLEIC (70%), SUGAR, LEMON JUICE, HONEY, DISTILLED VINEGAR, PAPRIKA, MUSTARD SEED, CELERY SEED

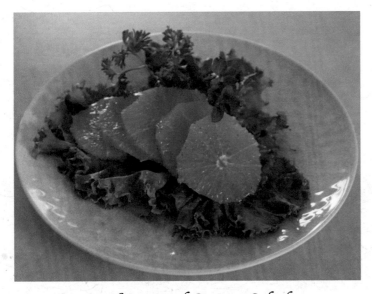

Honey and Orange Salad

Egg Salad

Serves 1

1 hard boiled egg
Leaf lettuce
1 Tbsp Thousand Island salad dressing

Place bed of lettuce on a plate. Arrange peeled, sliced hard boiled egg on lettuce. Drizzle salad dressing over egg. Serve.

Egg Salad

Nutrition Facts

1 serving per container

Serving size	**(200g)**

Amount Per Serving

Calories **150**

	% Daily Value*
Total Fat 11g	**14%**
Saturated Fat 2.5g	**13%**
Trans Fat 0g	
Cholesterol 190mg	**63%**
Sodium 230mg	**10%**
Total Carbohydrate 4g	**1%**
Dietary Fiber <1g	**3%**
Total Sugars 3g	
Includes 2g Added Sugars	**4%**
Protein 7g	
Vitamin D 1.1mcg	6%
Calcium 50mg	4%
Iron 1.2mg	6%
Potassium 170mg	4%

* The % Daily Value (DV) tells you how much a nutrient in a serving of food contributes to a daily diet. 2,000 calories a day is used for general nutrition advice.

INGREDIENTS: EGG, LETTUCE, SALAD DRESSING, THOUSAND ISLAND, COMMERCIAL, REGULAR

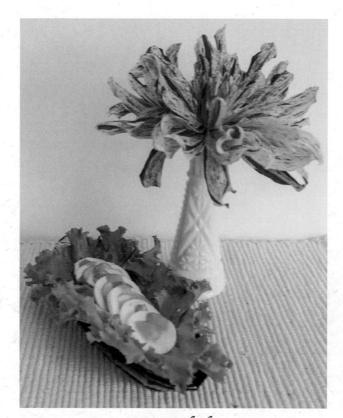

Egg Salad

Layered Fruit Salad

This makes a refreshing dessert or a very nice breakfast.

Serves 6

1 Tbsp lemon juice

1/4 cup honey

1/2 tsp grated orange peel

1/4 tsp ground cinnamon

2 cups peeled and sliced oranges

3 cups of fresh fruits (for nutritional guide 1 cup sweet cherries, 1 cup raspberries, 1 cup pineapple)

In a bowl, combine lemon juice, honey, orange peel and cinnamon. Add orange slices and toss to coat. Cover and chill overnight or for several hours. In serving dishes, layer some oranges on bottom. Layer other fruits on top. Drizzle with juice in bottom of bowl.

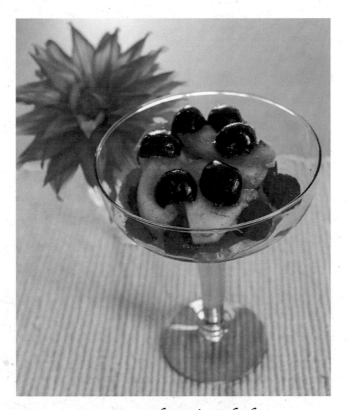

Layered Fruit Salad

Layered Fruit Salad

Nutrition Facts	
6 servings per container	
Serving size	**(152g)**

Amount Per Serving	
Calories	**110**

	% Daily Value*
Total Fat 0g	**0%**
Saturated Fat 0g	**0%**
Trans Fat 0g	
Cholesterol 0mg	**0%**
Sodium 0mg	**0%**
Total Carbohydrate 29g	**11%**
Dietary Fiber 4g	**14%**
Total Sugars 24g	
Includes 11g Added Sugars	**22%**
Protein 1g	
Vitamin D 0mcg	0%
Calcium 40mg	4%
Iron 0.4mg	2%
Potassium 240mg	6%

* The % Daily Value (DV) tells you how much a nutrient in a serving of food contributes to a daily diet. 2,000 calories a day is used for general nutrition advice.

INGREDIENTS: ORANGES, PINEAPPLE, CHERRIES, RASPBERRIES, HONEY, LEMON JUICE, CINNAMON, ORANGE ZEST

Carrot Raisin Salad

Serves 8 as a side dish

5 large carrots, peeled and shredded

1/2 cup raisins

1 cup thinly sliced celery

1/2 cup thinly sliced green onions

4 Tbsp sour cream

4 Tbsp Miracle Whip™

1 Tbsp lemon juice

Pepper to taste

Mix ingredients together, chill and serve.

Carrot-Raisin Salad

Nutrition Facts

8 servings per container

Serving size	(67g)

Amount Per Serving

Calories	45

% Daily Value*

Total Fat 2g	3%
Saturated Fat 0.5g	3%
Trans Fat 1g	
Cholesterol <5mg	1%
Sodium 95mg	4%
Total Carbohydrate 6g	2%
Dietary Fiber 1g	4%
Total Sugars 3g	
Includes 0g Added Sugars	0%
Protein 1g	
Vitamin D 0mcg	0%
Calcium 30mg	2%
Iron 0.2mg	2%
Potassium 170mg	4%

* The % Daily Value (DV) tells you how much a nutrient in a serving of food contributes to a daily diet. 2,000 calories a day is used for general nutrition advice.

INGREDIENTS: CARROTS, SOUR CREAM (CULTURED CREAM, SKIM MILK, VITAMIN A PALMITATE), SALAD DRESSING, KRAFT MIRACLE WHIP LIGHT DRESSING, GREEN ONIONS, LEMON JUICE, BLACK PEPPER

Chilled Strawberry Soup

This is the most requested menu item by my grandchildren when coming over. We gather and freeze strawberries when in season so they can have it all year round.

Serves 8

2 cups strawberries
1 cup apple juice
2/3 cup sugar
1 cup water - divided
1/2 tsp cinnamon
1/8 tsp cloves
16 oz strawberry yogurt

In a saucepan, combine apple juice, 3/4 cup water and spices. Bring to a boil. Cool. In a blender, puree strawberries and 1/4 cup water. Stir cooled apple juice mixture, strawberry mixture and yogurt until well blended. Chill and serve.

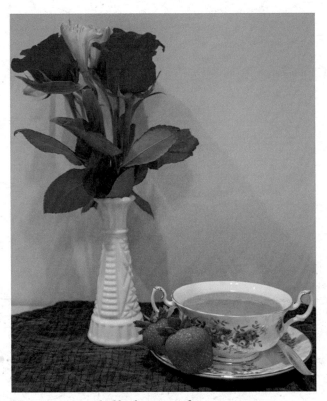

Chilled Strawberry Soup

Chilled Strawberry Soup

Nutrition Facts

8 servings per container

Serving size	**(178g)**

Amount Per Serving

Calories 160

	% Daily Value*
Total Fat 1.5g	**2%**
Saturated Fat 1g	**5%**
Trans Fat 0g	
Cholesterol 5mg	**2%**
Sodium 20mg	**1%**
Total Carbohydrate 32g	**12%**
Dietary Fiber 2g	**7%**
Total Sugars 30g	
Includes 23g Added Sugars	**46%**
Protein 5g	
Vitamin D 0mcg	0%
Calcium 60mg	4%
Iron 0.3mg	2%
Potassium 170mg	4%

* The % Daily Value (DV) tells you how much a nutrient in a serving of food contributes to a daily diet. 2,000 calories a day is used for general nutrition advice.

INGREDIENTS: YOGURT, GREEK, STRAWBERRY, LOWFAT, STRAWBERRIES, APPLE JUICE (APPLE JUICE, WATER, APPLE JUICE CONCENTRATE), WATER, SUGAR, CINNAMON, CLOVES

Cheese and Broccoli Soup

Serves 4

1 can no salt added cream of chicken soup

1 cup milk

2 cups shredded cheddar cheese

12 oz fresh broccoli, steamed

Combine all ingredients except cheese and heat until warm. Add cheese and cook until melted. Serve.

Cheese and Broccoli Soup

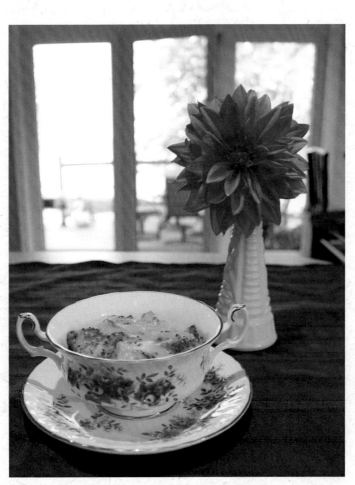

Cheese and Broccoli Soup

Nutrition Facts

4 servings per container

Serving size (270g)

Amount Per Serving

Calories **310**

	% Daily Value*
Total Fat 21g	**27%**
Saturated Fat 11g	**55%**
Trans Fat 0g	
Cholesterol 65mg	**22%**
Sodium 430mg	**19%**
Total Carbohydrate 13g	**5%**
Dietary Fiber 2g	**7%**
Total Sugars 4g	
Includes 0g Added Sugars	**0%**
Protein 19g	
Vitamin D 0.7mcg	4%
Calcium 510mg	40%
Iron 0.8mg	4%
Potassium 390mg	8%

* The % Daily Value (DV) tells you how much a nutrient in a serving of food contributes to a daily diet. 2,000 calories a day is used for general nutrition advice.

INGREDIENTS: BROCCOLI, MILK (PASTEURIZED REDUCED FAT MILK, VITAMIN A PALMITATE, VITAMIN D3), CHEDDAR (MILK, CULTURES, SALT, ENZYMES, ANNATTO (COLOR)), CHICKEN BROTH, MODIFIED CORN STARCH, WHEAT FLOUR, CHICKEN FAT, CHICKEN MEAT, VEGTABLE OIL, CREAM(MILK), YEAST EXTRACT, SOY PROTEIN ISOLATE, ONION POWDER, VINEGAR, BETA CAROTENE, FLAVOUR (CONTAINS CELERY)

Cauliflower Soup

Serves 8

1 medium peeled carrot shredded

1 medium head of cauliflower broken into florets

1/4 cup chopped celery

2 1/2 cups low sodium chicken broth

3 Tbsp unsalted butter

3 Tbsp all purpose flour

1/8 tsp pepper

2 cups milk

1 cup shredded cheddar cheese

In a large pot, combine cauliflower, carrot, celery and broth. Bring to a boil, cover and reduce heat. Simmer for 12-15 minutes until vegetables are tender. In another large saucepan, melt butter. Stir in flour and pepper. Cook until smooth. Gradually add milk. Bring to a boil over medium heat. Cook and stir for 2 minutes until thickened. Reduce heat and stir in cheese until melted. Stir into cauliflower and broth mixture.

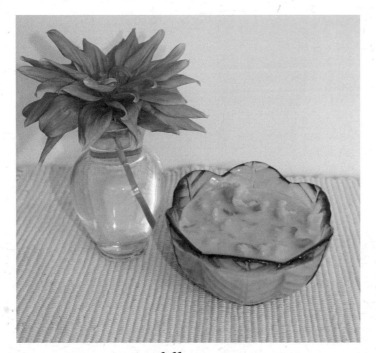

Cauliflower Soup

Cauliflower Soup

Nutrition Facts	
8 servings per container	
Serving size	**(246g)**

Amount Per Serving	
Calories	**190**

	% Daily Value*
Total Fat 10g	**13%**
Saturated Fat 6g	**30%**
Trans Fat 0g	
Cholesterol 35mg	**12%**
Sodium 180mg	**8%**
Total Carbohydrate 16g	**6%**
Dietary Fiber 2g	**7%**
Total Sugars 5g	
Includes 0g Added Sugars	**0%**
Protein 9g	
Vitamin D 0.7mcg	4%
Calcium 190mg	15%
Iron 0.8mg	4%
Potassium 400mg	8%

* The % Daily Value (DV) tells you how much a nutrient in a serving of food contributes to a daily diet. 2,000 calories a day is used for general nutrition advice.

INGREDIENTS: CAULIFLOWER, CAMPBELL'S LOW SODIUM SOUPS, CHICKEN BROTH, MILK (PASTEURIZED REDUCED FAT MILK, VITAMIN A PALMITATE, VITAMIN D3), CHEDDAR (MILK, CULTURES, SALT, ENZYMES, ANNATTO (COLOR)), ENRICHED UNBLEACHED FLOUR (WHEAT FLOUR, MALTED BARLEY FLOUR, NIACIN, IRON, THIAMINE, RIBOFLAVIN, FOLIC ACID), CARROTS, BUTTER (CREAM, NATURAL FLAVOR), CELERY, BLACK PEPPER

BEEF

1. Beef Enchiladas

2. Beef Tips in slow cooker

3. Beef Roll Ups

4. Beef Stroganoff

5. Porcupine Meatballs

6. Salisbury Steak

7. Ground Beef Dinner

8. Macaroni Meat

Beef Enchiladas

Serves 10

Preheat oven to 350°F

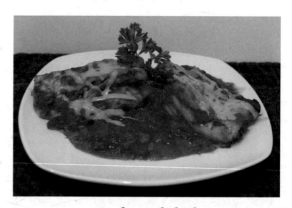

Beef Enchiladas

1 lb ground beef

1/2 cup chopped onion

1/2 cup chopped green pepper

1 clove minced garlic

1/2 cup whole kernel corn

1 (28 oz) can no salt added diced Italian tomatoes

1/2 tsp chili powder

1/2 tsp ground cumin

1 cup shredded cheddar cheese divided in half

1 small jar salsa

1 (15 oz) can no salt added tomato sauce

10 soft tortillas

In a skillet sauté onion, beef and garlic, stirring until meat is browned. Drain fat. Add tomatoes, green pepper, corn and spices. Reduce heat and simmer covered for 15 minutes.

Scoop equal amounts of mixture onto tortillas. Spread half of cheese over mixture amounts.

Spray a 9 x 13 baking dish (or two 8 x 8 baking dishes to freeze one for later) well with cooking spray then spread 3 Tbsp of tomato sauce on the bottom. Roll up tortillas and place in dish. Spread 2 Tbsp of tomato sauce and 2 Tbsp of salsa over each tortilla.

Bake covered for 20 minutes. Remove cover and sprinkle remaining cheese over tortillas. Bake for another 20 minutes.

Beef Enchiladas

Nutrition Facts

10 servings per container

Serving size	(0.0g)

Amount Per Serving

Calories **240**

	% Daily Value*
Total Fat 10g	13%
Saturated Fat 4.5g	23%
Trans Fat 0g	
Cholesterol 40mg	13%
Sodium 380mg	17%
Total Carbohydrate 22g	8%
Dietary Fiber 4g	14%
Total Sugars 6g	
Includes 0g Added Sugars	0%
Protein 15g	
Vitamin D 0mcg	0%
Calcium 170mg	15%
Iron 2.5mg	15%
Potassium 420mg	8%

* The % Daily Value (DV) tells you how much a nutrient in a serving of food contributes to a daily diet. 2,000 calories a day is used for general nutrition advice.

INGREDIENTS: DICED PLUM TOMATOES NO SALT ADDED, GROUND BEEF, TOMATO SAUCE (TOMATOES, TOMATO JUICE, <2% OF: SALT, CITRIC ACID, CALCIUM CHLORIDE), SAUCE, SALSA, READY-TO-SERVE, TORTILLA (CORN MASA FLOUR, WATER, CELLULOSE GUM, PROPIONIC ACID (TO PRESERVE FRESHNESS), BENZOIC ACID (TO PRESERVE FRESHNESS), PHOSPHORIC ACID (PRESERVATIVE), GUAR GUM, AMYLASE), CHEDDAR (MILK, CULTURES, SALT, ENZYMES, ANNATTO (COLOR)), ONIONS, GREEN PEPPERS, CORN, GARLIC, CHILI POWDER, SALT-FREE, CUMIN

Beef Tips in Slow Cooker

Serves 4

8 oz sliced mushrooms

1 small onion sliced

1 Tbsp olive oil

1 lb stew beef cut into one-inch cubes

1 Tbsp Worcestershire sauce

1/2 cup red wine (alcoholic or non-alcoholic)

2 1/2 cups low sodium beef broth

2 Tbsp corn starch

1/4 cup cold water

Place the onions and mushrooms into the bottom of a 4.5 quart slow cooker. Heat the oil in a skillet over medium-high heat. Add beef and sear on all sides. Do not cook through. Place meat in slow cooker on top of the vegetables. Add 2 Tbsp of red wine to skillet, scraping bits off bottom and then add to slow cooker. Add Worcestershire sauce and balance of red wine and beef broth to slow cooker. Cover and cook on low for 6-8 hours. Whisk corn starch and cold water together. Whisk into slow cooker. Cover and cook on high for another 45 minutes.

Serve over egg noodles, mashed potatoes or rice.

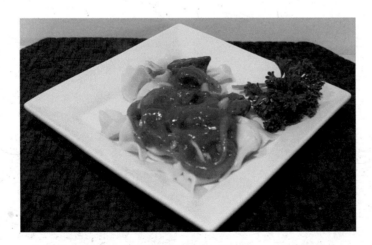

Beef Tips

Beef Tips

Nutrition Facts	
4 servings per container	
Serving size	**(0.0g)**

Amount Per Serving	
Calories	**230**

	% Daily Value*
Total Fat 9g	**12%**
Saturated Fat 2.5g	**13%**
Trans Fat 0g	
Cholesterol 70mg	**23%**
Sodium 140mg	**6%**
Total Carbohydrate 6g	**2%**
Dietary Fiber 0g	**0%**
Total Sugars 1g	
Includes 0g Added Sugars	**0%**
Protein 25g	
Vitamin D 0.1mcg	0%
Calcium 20mg	2%
Iron 2.8mg	15%
Potassium 550mg	10%

*The % Daily Value (DV) tells you how much a nutrient in a serving of food contributes to a daily diet. 2,000 calories a day is used for general nutrition advice.

INGREDIENTS: BEEF, BEEF STOCK, WATER, YEAST EXTRACT, DEXTROSE, SUGAR, ONION JUICE CONCENTRATE, TOMATO PASTE, BEEF FAT, NATURAL FLAVOUR (CONTAINS CELERY, GARLIC), RED WINE, MUSHROOMS, WATER, WORCESTERSHIRE SAUCE (DISTILLED WHITE VINEGAR, ANCHOVIES, GARLIC, MOLASSES, ONIONS, SALT, SUGAR, WATER, CHILI PEPPER EXTRACT, CLOVES, NATURAL FLAVORINGS, TAMARIND EXTRACT), CORNSTARCH, OLIVE OIL, ONION

Beef Roll Ups

Serves 6

1 1/2 lb round steak (have the meat dept. or butcher shop run it through the meat tenderizer)

1/4 cup chopped onion

1/2 cup chopped celery

2 cups fresh bread cubes

1/4 cup unsalted butter (melted)

1 Tbsp dried parsley flakes

1/2 tsp poultry seasoning

1/4 tsp pepper

1 cup flour

2 Tbsp cooking oil

1 can no salt added mushroom soup

1 1/3 cups water

Cut steak into 6 pieces, keeping in mind you are stuffing and rolling them up. Combine next seven ingredients and put equal amounts on each steak piece. Roll up and hold with tooth picks. Roll in flour. Brown in oil in a large skillet. Whisk soup and water together. Pour over steak roll ups and simmer for two hours or until meat is tender, turning occasionally.

Beef Roll Ups

Nutrition Facts

6 servings per container

Serving size	**1 (0.0g)**

Amount Per Serving

Calories — **310**

	% Daily Value*
Total Fat 12g	**15%**
Saturated Fat 3.5g	**18%**
Trans Fat 0g	
Cholesterol 75mg	**25%**
Sodium 90mg	**4%**
Total Carbohydrate 20g	**7%**
Dietary Fiber <1g	**3%**
Total Sugars <1g	
Includes 0g Added Sugars	**0%**
Protein 28g	
Vitamin D 0mcg	0%
Calcium 30mg	2%
Iron 4.6mg	25%
Potassium 490mg	10%

* The % Daily Value (DV) tells you how much a nutrient in a serving of food contributes to a daily diet. 2,000 calories a day is used for general nutrition advice.

INGREDIENTS: BEEF, ROUND, OUTSIDE ROUND, BOTTOM ROUND, STEAK, SEPARABLE LEAN AND FAT, TRIMMED TO 0" FAT, SELECT, RAW, WATER, WATER, MUSHROOMS, VEGETABLE OIL, MODIFIED CORN STARCH, WHEAT FLOUR, CREAM (MILK), WHEY POWDER, SOY PROTEIN ISOLATE, TOMATO PASTE, SPICE EXTRACT, YEAST EXTRACT, DEHYDRATED GARLIC FLAVOUR, ENRICHED BLEACHED FLOUR (WHEAT FLOUR, MALTED BARLEY FLOUR, NIACIN, IRON, THIAMINE, RIBOFLAVIN, FOLIC ACID), CELERY, ONIONS, BUTTER (CREAM, NATURAL FLAVOR), CANOLA VEGETABLE OIL, POULTRY SEASONING (THYME, SAGE, MARJORAM, ROSEMARY, BLACK PEPPER, AND NUTMEG), BLACK PEPPER, PARSLEY

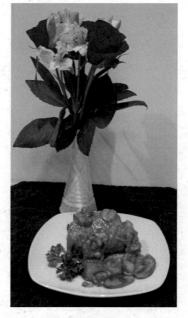

Beef Roll Ups

Beef Stroganoff

Serves 6

3 Tbsp unsalted butter

1 1/2 lb one-inch stew beef cubes

1/2 tsp pepper

2 Tbsp flour

2 cups half and half cream

3 oz cream cheese softened

2 Tbsp tomato paste

2 cups mushrooms sliced

1 cup pearl onions

1/2 cup chopped fresh parsley

1 tsp marjoram leaves

Melt butter in a skillet. Add beef and pepper, cooking over medium high heat until browned. Stir in flour and toss to coat steak. Add cream, tomato paste and cream cheese. Reduce heat to medium, cooking and stirring until sauce is thickened (approximately 8 minutes). Stir in remaining ingredients. Continue cooking approximately 4 minutes until onions and mushrooms are tender. Serve over cooked egg noodles.

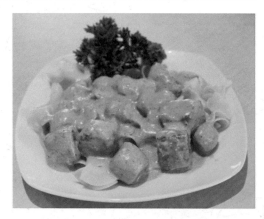

Beef Stroganoff

Beef Stroganoff

Nutrition Facts	
6 servings per container	
Serving size	**(0.0g)**

Amount Per Serving	
Calories	**460**

	% Daily Value*
Total Fat 24g	**31%**
Saturated Fat 14g	**70%**
Trans Fat 1g	
Cholesterol 130mg	**43%**
Sodium 190mg	**8%**
Total Carbohydrate 30g	**11%**
Dietary Fiber 4g	**14%**
Total Sugars 13g	
Includes 0g Added Sugars	**0%**
Protein 32g	
Vitamin D 0.2mcg	0%
Calcium 130mg	10%
Iron 3.3mg	20%
Potassium 710mg	15%

* The % Daily Value (DV) tells you how much a nutrient in a serving of food contributes to a daily diet. 2,000 calories a day is used for general nutrition advice.

INGREDIENTS: BEEF, HALF AND HALF (MILK, CREAM), PEARL ONIONS, MUSHROOMS, CREAM CHEESE (MILK, CHEESE CULTURES, SALT, GUAR GUM), BUTTER (CREAM, NATURAL FLAVOR), TOMATO PASTE (TOMATOES), PARSLEY, ENRICHED BLEACHED FLOUR (WHEAT FLOUR, MALTED BARLEY FLOUR, NIACIN, IRON, THIAMINE, RIBOFLAVIN, FOLIC ACID), BLACK PEPPER, MARJORAM

Porcupine Meatballs

One of our daughter's favourites.

Serves 4

Preheat oven to 375°F

Meatballs

1/2 tsp pepper
1/2 tsp basil leaves
1/2 cup water
1/2 cup uncooked long grain rice
1 lb ground beef

Sauce

1 tsp minced garlic
1/4 tsp pepper
1 (6 oz) can low sodium tomato paste
1 medium onion chopped
2 stalks celery chopped
3 medium tomatoes cut into 1-inch pieces
1 cup water

Mix all meatball ingredients together in a medium bowl. Form 12 meatballs and place in an 8 x 12 baking dish. Mix all sauce ingredients in a medium bowl. Pour over meatballs. Cover and bake for 45-50 minutes.

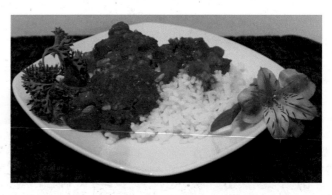

Porcupine Meatballs

Porcupine Meatballs

Nutrition Facts	
4 servings per container	
Serving size	**(0.0g)**
Amount Per Serving	
Calories	**400**
	% Daily Value*
Total Fat 17g	**22%**
Saturated Fat 7g	**35%**
Trans Fat 1g	
Cholesterol 75mg	**25%**
Sodium 130mg	**6%**
Total Carbohydrate 35g	**13%**
Dietary Fiber 5g	**18%**
Total Sugars 9g	
Includes 0g Added Sugars	**0%**
Protein 25g	
Vitamin D 0.1mcg	0%
Calcium 50mg	4%
Iron 5.7mg	30%
Potassium 1110mg	25%

* The % Daily Value (DV) tells you how much a nutrient in a serving of food contributes to a daily diet. 2,000 calories a day is used for general nutrition advice.

INGREDIENTS: GROUND BEEF, TOMATOES, WATER, TOMATO PASTE (TOMATOES), ONION, RICE, WHITE, LONG-GRAIN, REGULAR, RAW, ENRICHED, CELERY, GARLIC, BLACK PEPPER, BASIL

Salisbury Steak

Serves 4

1 lb ground beef

1/3 cup fresh bread crumbs

1 large egg

1 Tbsp Worcestershire sauce

1 Tbsp ketchup

1 minced garlic clove

Pepper

1 Tbsp olive oil

Gravy Ingredients

2 Tbsp unsalted butter

1 chopped onion

1/2 tsp thyme

1/2 cup thinly sliced mushrooms

2 Tbsp flour

1 Tbsp Worcestershire sauce

1 Tbsp (1% sodium) tomato paste

1 cup no sodium added beef stock

Pepper

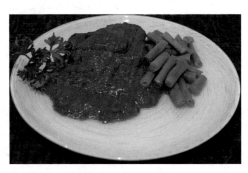

Salisbury Steak

Salisbury Steak

Nutrition Facts	
4 servings per container	
Serving size	**(0.0g)**
Amount Per Serving	
Calories	**430**
	% Daily Value*
Total Fat 28g	36%
Saturated Fat 11g	55%
Trans Fat 1g	
Cholesterol 140mg	47%
Sodium 320mg	14%
Total Carbohydrate 17g	6%
Dietary Fiber 1g	4%
Total Sugars 5g	
Includes 1g Added Sugars	2%
Protein 25g	
Vitamin D 0.4mcg	2%
Calcium 70mg	6%
Iron 4.2mg	25%
Potassium 570mg	10%

* The % Daily Value (DV) tells you how much a nutrient in a serving of food contributes to a daily diet. 2,000 calories a day is used for general nutrition advice.

INGREDIENTS: GROUND BEEF, BEEF STOCK, WATER, YEAST EXTRACT, DEXTROSE, SUGAR, ONION JUICE CONCENTRATE, TOMATO PASTE, BEEF FAT, NATURAL FLAVOUR (CONTAINS CELERY, GARLIC), ONION, WHITE BREAD (ENRICHED WHEAT FLOUR (FLOUR, MALTED BARLEY FLOUR, NIACIN, IRON (FERROUS SULFATE, REDUCED IRON), THIAMINE MONONITRATE, RIBOFLAVIN, FOLIC ACID), WATER, YEAST, SALT, SOYBEAN OIL, SUGAR, MALT, DOUGH CONDITIONERS (ASCORBIC ACID, CALCIUM SULFATE, SODIUM STEAROYL LACTYLATE), CALCIUM PROPIONATE (PRESERVATIVE)), EGG, MUSHROOMS, WORCESTERSHIRE SAUCE (DISTILLED WHITE VINEGAR, ANCHOVIES, GARLIC, MOLASSES, ONIONS, SALT, SUGAR, WATER, CHILI PEPPER EXTRACT, CLOVES, NATURAL FLAVORINGS, TAMARIND EXTRACT), BUTTER (CREAM, NATURAL FLAVOR), TOMATO PASTE (TOMATOES), KETCHUP (TOMATO CONCENTRATE FROM RED RIPE TOMATOES, DISTILLED VINEGAR, HIGH FRUCTOSE CORN SYRUP, CORN SYRUP, SALT, SPICE, ONION POWDER, NATURAL FLAVORING), OLIVE OIL, GARLIC, ENRICHED UNBLEACHED FLOUR (WHEAT FLOUR, MALTED BARLEY FLOUR, NIACIN, IRON, THIAMINE, RIBOFLAVIN, FOLIC ACID), BLACK PEPPER, THYME

Combine patty ingredients in a large bowl and form four patties.

In a large skillet over medium heat, heat oil and sear both sides of patties (approximately 5 minutes per side). Remove from pan.

Wipe out skillet and add butter. Add onions and thyme and stir until onions are soft. Add mushrooms and cook until browned and tender, approximately 4 minutes. Sprinkle with flour and stir until coated. Cook for another 2 minutes. Add Worcestershire sauce, tomato paste, pepper and beef stock. Bring to a simmer and return patties to skillet. Cover and cook for 10 - 15 minutes until patties are done and the sauce has thickened.

Ground Beef Dinner

This is a simple weeknight meal when you don't have a lot of time.

Serves 4

Preheat oven to 400°F

1 lb ground beef
3-4 medium potatoes peeled and sliced
3 medium carrots peeled and sliced
1 onion peeled and sliced
Pepper

Combine all ingredients in a roast pan. Pepper to taste.
Bake for 20-30 minutes until cooked.

Ground Beef Dinner

Nutrition Facts	
4 servings per container	
Serving size	**(0.0g)**

Amount Per Serving	
Calories	**420**

	% Daily Value*
Total Fat 17g	**22%**
Saturated Fat 7g	**35%**
Trans Fat 1g	
Cholesterol 75mg	**25%**
Sodium 140mg	**6%**
Total Carbohydrate 41g	**15%**
Dietary Fiber 7g	**25%**
Total Sugars 6g	
Includes 0g Added Sugars	**0%**
Protein 25g	
Vitamin D 0.1mcg	0%
Calcium 60mg	4%
Iron 3.7mg	20%
Potassium 1390mg	30%

* The % Daily Value (DV) tells you how much a nutrient in a serving of food contributes to a daily diet. 2,000 calories a day is used for general nutrition advice.

INGREDIENTS: POTATOES, GROUND BEEF, CARROTS, ONION, BLACK PEPPER

Macaroni Meat

Serves 4

1 lb ground beef
1 can of tomato soup
2 cups elbow macaroni cooked as per instructions
1 slice cheddar cheese

Cook macaroni as per instructions. Set aside. Sauté ground beef in a frying pan. Add macaroni to beef and mix in tomato soup. Cook until heated through. Break up cheese and place on top of mixture. When melted, stir in. Serve.

Macaroni Meat

Nutrition Facts

Serving Size: (216g)
Servings Per Container: 4

Amount Per Serving

Calories 410   Calories from Fat 170

% Daily Value*

Total Fat 19g	**29%**
Saturated Fat 7g	**35%**
Trans Fat 1g	
Cholesterol 80mg	**27%**
Sodium 360mg	**15%**
Total Carbohydrate 31g	**10%**
Dietary Fiber 2g	**8%**
Sugars 7g	
Protein 27g	

Vitamin A 6%	•	Vitamin C 6%	
Calcium 6%	•	Iron 20%	

* Percent Daily Values are based on a 2,000 calorie diet. Your daily values may be higher or lower depending on your calorie needs:

		Calories:	2,000	2,500
Total Fat	Less than		65g	80g
Sat Fat	Less than		20g	25g
Cholesterol	Less than		300mg	300mg
Sodium	Less than		2,400mg	2,400mg
Total Carbohydrate			300g	375g
Dietary Fiber			25g	30g

INGREDIENTS: GROUND BEEF, CAMPBELL'S, TOMATO SOUP, CONDENSED, SEMOLINA WHEAT, DURUM WHEAT FLOUR, VITAMIN B3 NIACIN, IRON FERROUS SULFATE, VITAMIN B1 THIAMINE MONONITRATE, VITAMIN B2 RIBOFLAVIN, FOLIC ACID., CHEESE, CHEDDAR, SHARP, SLICED

CHICKEN

1. Chicken Alfredo

2. Chicken Enchiladas

3. Chicken/Turkey Pot Pie

4. Grilled Chicken with Lemon Asparagus Pasta

5. Saucy French Onion Chicken

6. Tomato Basil Chicken

Chicken Alfredo

Serves 4

Preheat oven to 350°F

2 cups cooked shredded chicken

8 cooked lasagne noodles

3 Tbsp unsalted butter

2 minced garlic cloves

3 Tbsp flour

2 1/4 cups milk

1/2 cup grated low sodium Parmesan cheese

2 Tbsp softened cream cheese

Juice of 1/2 lemon

2 tsp chopped parsley, divided

Pepper

Butter a large casserole dish. Melt butter in a skillet (medium heat), add garlic and sauté approximately 1 to 1 1/2 minutes. Whisk in flour, stirring until bubbly. Add milk slowly, stirring. Bring to simmer and stir in cream cheese and Parmesan. Continue stirring for 2-3 minutes until sauce thickens. Add lemon juice and 1 tsp parsley. Divide sauce in half. Season one half of sauce with pepper and stir in the chicken. Set aside. Divide other half of sauce. Spread half on bottom of casserole dish. Set aside remaining sauce.

Lay cooked lasagne noodles on flat surface. Spread chicken Alfredo mixture on each noodle and roll up. Lay roll ups in casserole dish. Cover with remaining sauce. Sprinkle with remaining parsley. Bake uncovered for 20 minutes.

NOTE: You can use other noodles and place in sauce with chunks of chicken and cooked vegetables.

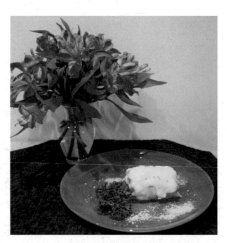

Chicken Alfredo

Chicken Alfredo

Nutrition Facts		
4 servings per container		
Serving size		**(0.0g)**
Amount Per Serving		
Calories		**470**
		% Daily Value*
Total Fat 21g		27%
Saturated Fat 12g		60%
Trans Fat 0g		
Cholesterol 170mg		57%
Sodium 160mg		7%
Total Carbohydrate 23g		8%
Dietary Fiber <1g		2%
Total Sugars 7g		
Includes 0g Added Sugars		0%
Protein 47g		
Vitamin D 1.8mcg		8%
Calcium 280mg		20%
Iron 1.4mg		8%
Potassium 690mg		15%

* The % Daily Value (DV) tells you how much a nutrient in a serving of food contributes to a daily diet. 2,000 calories a day is used for general nutrition advice.

INGREDIENTS: MILK (PASTEURIZED REDUCED FAT MILK, VITAMIN A PALMITATE, VITAMIN D3), CHICKEN, WHOLE-GRAIN BROWN RICE (RICE BRAN), CHEESE, PARMESAN, LOW SODIUM, ENRICHED UNBLEACHED FLOUR (WHEAT FLOUR, MALTED BARLEY FLOUR, NIACIN, IRON, THIAMINE, RIBOFLAVIN, FOLIC ACID), BUTTER (CREAM, NATURAL FLAVOR), CREAM CHEESE (MILK, CHEESE CULTURES, SALT, GUAR GUM), LEMON JUICE, GARLIC, PARSLEY, BLACK PEPPER

Chicken Enchiladas

Serves 10

Preheat oven to 350 °F

8 oz sour cream

1/2 cup onion, chopped

1 large bottle salsa

2 cups cooked chicken, chopped

1 cup shredded cheese, divided

2-4 minced garlic cloves

1 tsp cumin

10 small tortillas

I divide into two baking dishes to freeze one for a later date. Use either a 9 x 13 inch baking dish or two 8 x 8 baking dishes.

Combine sour cream, onion, chicken, 1/2 cup cheese, garlic and cumin in a bowl. Mix well. Spread 4 Tbsp salsa on bottom of baking dish. Spoon chicken mixture into tortillas and roll up. Place in baking dish. Cover each tortilla with approximately 4 Tbsp salsa. Cover and bake for 30 minutes. Sprinkle with remaining cheese. Bake uncovered for another 30 minutes.

Chicken Enchiladas

Nutrition Facts	
10 servings per container	
Serving size	**(0.0g)**

Amount Per Serving	
Calories	**240**

	% Daily Value*
Total Fat 9g	**12%**
Saturated Fat 4g	**20%**
Trans Fat 0g	
Cholesterol 65mg	**22%**
Sodium 910mg	**40%**
Total Carbohydrate 21g	**8%**
Dietary Fiber 3g	**11%**
Total Sugars 5g	
Includes 0g Added Sugars	**0%**
Protein 21g	
Vitamin D 0.1mcg	0%
Calcium 190mg	15%
Iron 1.1mg	6%
Potassium 450mg	10%

* The % Daily Value (DV) tells you how much a nutrient in a serving of food contributes to a daily diet. 2,000 calories a day is used for general nutrition advice.

INGREDIENTS: SAUCE, SALSA, READY-TO-SERVE, CHICKEN, MISSION FOODS, MISSION FLOUR TORTILLAS, SOFT TACO, 8 INCH, SOUR CREAM (CULTURED CREAM, SKIM MILK, VITAMIN A PALMITATE), CHEDDAR (MILK, CULTURES, SALT, ENZYMES, ANNATTO (COLOR)), ONIONS, GARLIC, CUMIN

Chicken/Turkey Pot Pie

Serves 8

Preheat oven to 400°F

1 can no salt added cream of mushroom soup

5 oz evaporated milk

1/2 tsp dried thyme

1/4 cup minced fresh parsley

3 cups cubed cooked chicken or turkey

1 small package frozen mixed vegetable

1/4 tsp pepper

6-8 potatoes

1/2 cup milk

Paprika (optional)

Peel, boil and mash potatoes with milk. Set aside. In a bowl, combine the rest of ingredients. Grease an 11 x 7 baking pan and spoon chicken/turkey mixture into it. Spread mashed potatoes over top. Sprinkle with paprika (optional). Bake uncovered for 20-30 minutes.

Chicken/Turkey Pot Pie

Nutrition Facts

8 servings per container

Serving size	(403g)

Amount Per Serving

Calories 360

	% Daily Value*
Total Fat 6g	8%
Saturated Fat 2g	10%
Trans Fat 0g	
Cholesterol 75mg	25%
Sodium 170mg	7%
Total Carbohydrate 43g	16%
Dietary Fiber 7g	25%
Total Sugars 7g	
Includes 0g Added Sugars	0%
Protein 33g	
Vitamin D 0.8mcg	4%
Calcium 110mg	8%
Iron 2.4mg	15%
Potassium 1270mg	25%

* The % Daily Value (DV) tells you how much a nutrient in a serving of food contributes to a daily diet. 2,000 calories a day is used for general nutrition advice.

INGREDIENTS: POTATOES, TURKEY BREAST (TURKEY BREAST, TURKEY BROTH, CONTAINS 2% OR LESS OF DEXTROSE, MODIFIED FOOD STARCH, SALT, VINEGAR, SODIUM PHOSPHATE), MIXED VEGETABLES (PEAS, CARROTS, GREEN BEANS, CORN), WATER, MUSHROOMS, VEGETABLE OIL, MODIFIED CORN STARCH, WHEAT FLOUR, CREAM (MILK), WHEY POWDER, SOY PROTEIN ISOLATE, TOMATO PASTE, SPICE EXTRACT, YEAST EXTRACT, DEHYDRATED GARLIC FLAVOUR, 'NESTLE CARNATION' EVAPORATED MILK (VITAMIN D ADDED), MILK (PASTEURIZED REDUCED FAT MILK, VITAMIN A PALMITATE, VITAMIN D3), PARSLEY, BLACK PEPPER, THYME

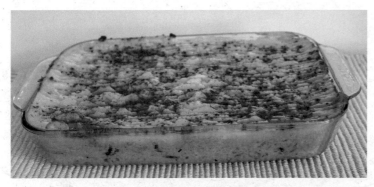

Chicken/Turkey Pot Pie

Grilled Chicken with Lemon Asparagus Pasta

Serves 4

4 small boneless, skinless chicken breasts, grilled and cut into strips

4 servings pasta (penne, linguine, etc.)

1 lb asparagus cut into 1-inch pieces

3/4 cup heavy cream

2 Tbsp unsalted butter

1/2 tsp pepper

1/2 Tbsp fresh lemon zest

1/2 Tbsp fresh lemon juice

1/3 cup fresh grated Parmesan cheese

Cook pasta in water as per package instructions. Add asparagus to pot during last 3 minutes. Drain, reserving 1/4 cup of liquid.

In a small pot, combine heavy cream, butter and pepper. Cook over medium-high heat and simmer until thick enough to coat a spoon (approximately 4 minutes). Remove from heat and stir in lemon juice and zest. Add pasta and vegetables, toss to coat. Add pasta water if it needs thinning. Arrange chicken slices on plate and add pasta and vegetables in sauce.

Grilled Chicken with Lemon Asparagus Pasta

Nutrition Facts

4 servings per container

Serving size	(266g)

Amount Per Serving

Calories	470

	% Daily Value*
Total Fat 19g	24%
Saturated Fat 10g	50%
Trans Fat 0g	
Cholesterol 105mg	35%
Sodium 200mg	9%
Total Carbohydrate 48g	17%
Dietary Fiber 8g	29%
Total Sugars 4g	
Includes 0g Added Sugars	0%
Protein 30g	
Vitamin D 0.4mcg	2%
Calcium 110mg	8%
Iron 3.2mg	20%
Potassium 520mg	10%

* The % Daily Value (DV) tells you how much a nutrient in a serving of food contributes to a daily diet. 2,000 calories a day is used for general nutrition advice.

INGREDIENTS: ASPARAGUS, CHICKEN, PASTA (WHOLE WHEAT FLOUR), HEAVY CREAM (HEAVY CREAM, SKIM MILK, CARRAGEENAN), PARMESAN (MILK, CHEESE CULTURES, SALT, ENZYMES), BUTTER (CREAM, NATURAL FLAVOR), LEMON JUICE, LEMON PEEL, BLACK PEPPER

Saucy French Onion Chicken

Serves 4

Preheat oven to 400°F

2 medium onions thinly sliced into rings

3 Tbsp unsalted butter

4 small boneless skinless chicken breasts

1 Tbsp oil

1 cup plus 3 Tbsp low sodium beef broth divided

Pepper to taste

1 tsp Italian seasoning

2 Tbsp flour

4 slices provolone cheese

4 slices of Swiss cheese

1/4 cup shredded Parmesan cheese

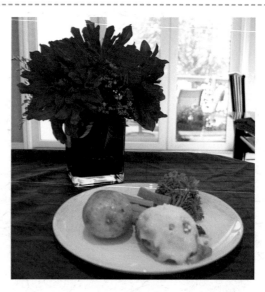

Saucy French Onion Chicken

In a large skillet over medium high heat, sauté butter, onions and 3 Tbsp beef broth 15-18 minutes, stirring and adjusting heat if necessary, until very browned and tender. Keep warm in a separate bowl. In same pan, cook chicken by drizzling with oil and seasoning with pepper and Italian seasoning. Cook 4-5 minutes on each side until browned. Put on a separate plate. Return onions to pan, sprinkle with flour and stir for 1 minute over medium heat. Add remaining beef broth and continue to cook, stirring until mixture comes to a boil. Transfer onion mixture into a baking dish. Add chicken and spoon sauce over chicken. Place one slice of provolone cheese and then one slice of Swiss cheese over each piece of chicken. Sprinkle with Parmesan cheese. Bake in oven for 10 minutes until chicken is cooked through and cheeses are melted.

Saucy French Onion Chicken

Nutrition Facts

4 servings per container

Serving size	**(327g)**

Amount Per Serving

Calories 530

	% Daily Value*
Total Fat 31g	**40%**
Saturated Fat 16g	**80%**
Trans Fat 0.5g	
Cholesterol 185mg	**62%**
Sodium 540mg	**23%**
Total Carbohydrate 10g	**4%**
Dietary Fiber 1g	**4%**
Total Sugars 3g	
Includes 0g Added Sugars	**0%**
Protein 52g	
Vitamin D 0.2mcg	2%
Calcium 530mg	40%
Iron 1.2mg	6%
Potassium 590mg	15%

* The % Daily Value (DV) tells you how much a nutrient in a serving of food contributes to a daily diet. 2,000 calories a day is used for general nutrition advice.

INGREDIENTS: CHICKEN, BEEF STOCK, WATER, YEAST EXTRACT, DEXTROSE, SUGAR, ONION JUICE CONCENTRATE, TOMATO PASTE, BEEF FAT, NATURAL FLAVOUR (CONTAINS CELERY, GARLIC), ONION, PROVOLONE (PASTEURIZED MILK, CHEESE CULTURE, SALT, ENZYMES), SWISS CHEESE (PASTEURIZED PART-SKIM MILK, CHEESE CULTURES, SALT, ENZYMES), PARMESAN (MILK, CHEESE CULTURES, SALT, ENZYMES), BUTTER (CREAM, NATURAL FLAVOR), ENRICHED BLEACHED FLOUR (WHEAT FLOUR, MALTED BARLEY FLOUR, NIACIN, IRON, THIAMINE, RIBOFLAVIN, FOLIC ACID), OIL, VEGETABLE, NATREON CANOLA, HIGH STABILITY, NON TRANS, HIGH OLEIC (70%), BLACK PEPPER, OREGANO, BASIL

Tomato Basil Chicken

This is one of my favourite recipes. Fresh basil and breadcrumbs make all the difference in the flavour of this recipe.

Serves 6

Preheat oven to 350°F

Sauce Ingredients

3 Tbsp unsalted butter

2 cups 1-inch cubed ripe tomatoes

1/3 cup chopped onion

1 (6 oz) can 1% sodium tomato paste

3 Tbsp chopped fresh basil leaves

1/4 tsp pepper

1 tsp minced garlic

3 boneless, skinless chicken breasts, halved

Topping

1 cup fresh breadcrumbs

1/4 cup chopped fresh parsley

1 Tbsp melted unsalted butter

3/4 cup shredded mozzarella cheese

Melt 3 Tbsp butter in 9 x 13 baking dish in the oven. Add chicken, toss to coat. In a medium bowl, stir together remaining sauce ingredients. Spoon sauce mixture over chicken. Bake for 30-40 minutes until chicken is cooked through. While waiting, mix all topping ingredients in bowl except cheese. Sprinkle mozzarella cheese over chicken when done. Sprinkle topping mixture on top of cheese and bake for 5-10 minutes longer until breadcrumbs are browned.

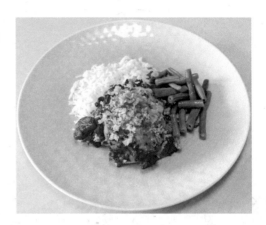

Tomato Basil Chicken

Tomato Basil Chicken

Nutrition Facts		
6 servings per container		
Serving size		**(216g)**
Amount Per Serving		
Calories		**330**
		% Daily Value*
Total Fat 13g		17%
Saturated Fat 7g		35%
Trans Fat 0g		
Cholesterol 85mg		28%
Sodium 310mg		13%
Total Carbohydrate 29g		11%
Dietary Fiber 4g		14%
Total Sugars 8g		
Includes 0g Added Sugars		0%
Protein 25g		
Vitamin D 0.1mcg		0%
Calcium 150mg		10%
Iron 3.3mg		20%
Potassium 730mg		15%

* The % Daily Value (DV) tells you how much a nutrient in a serving of food contributes to a daily diet. 2,000 calories a day is used for general nutrition advice.

INGREDIENTS: TOMATOES, CHICKEN, WHITE BREAD (ENRICHED WHEAT FLOUR (FLOUR, MALTED BARLEY FLOUR, NIACIN, IRON (FERROUS SULFATE, REDUCED IRON), THIAMINE MONONITRATE, RIBOFLAVIN, FOLIC ACID), WATER, YEAST, SALT, SOYBEAN OIL, SUGAR, MALT, DOUGH CONDITIONERS (ASCORBIC ACID, CALCIUM SULFATE, SODIUM STEAROYL LACTYLATE), CALCIUM PROPIONATE (PRESERVATIVE)), TOMATO PASTE (TOMATOES), CHEESE, MOZZARELLA, LOW MOISTURE, PART-SKIM, SHREDDED, BUTTER (CREAM, NATURAL FLAVOR), ONIONS, PARSLEY, BASIL, GARLIC, BLACK PEPPER

MISCELLANEOUS

1. Macaroni & Cheese

2. Manicotti

3. Moon Chilli

4. Pancake Batter

5. Pasta Sauce

6. Potatoes Romanoff

7. Scalloped Potatoes

8. Sunshine Jam

Macaroni and Cheese

One of my picky eater grandsons helped me make this and ate two platefuls. Now he says he loves it!

Serves 8

Preheat oven to 400°F

2 cups elbow macaroni cooked as per package instructions

1/4 cup unsalted butter

3 Tbsp flour

2 cups milk

1 (8 oz) package cream cheese, softened

1/2 tsp pepper

2 tsp Dijon mustard

2 cups shredded cheddar cheese

Topping

1 cup fresh breadcrumbs

2 Tbsp unsalted butter, melted

2 Tbsp chopped fresh parsley (or 2 tsp dried parsley)

In a 3-quart saucepan, melt butter. Stir in flour and cook until bubbly (1 minute). Stir in milk, cream cheese, pepper and cook until cheese is melted. Add mustard and cheddar cheese and stir. Pour into a 2-quart casserole dish. Stir in macaroni. In a small bowl, mix topping ingredients and sprinkle over macaroni and cheese. Bake for 15-20 minutes until heated through.

Macaroni & Cheese

Nutrition Facts

8 servings per container

Serving size	(284g)

Amount Per Serving

Calories	810

	% Daily Value*
Total Fat 31g	**40%**
Saturated Fat 17g	**85%**
Trans Fat 0g	
Cholesterol 95mg	**32%**
Sodium 480mg	**21%**
Total Carbohydrate 107g	**39%**
Dietary Fiber 5g	**18%**
Total Sugars 10g	
Includes 0g Added Sugars	**0%**
Protein 28g	
Vitamin D 0.7mcg	4%
Calcium 340mg	25%
Iron 5mg	30%
Potassium 140mg	2%

* The % Daily Value (DV) tells you how much a nutrient in a serving of food contributes to a daily diet. 2,000 calories a day is used for general nutrition advice.

INGREDIENTS: SEMOLINA WHEAT, DURUM WHEAT FLOUR, VITAMIN B3 NIACIN, IRON FERROUS SULFATE, VITAMIN B1 THIAMINE MONONITRATE, VITAMIN B2 RIBOFLAVIN, FOLIC ACID., MILK (PASTEURIZED REDUCED FAT MILK, VITAMIN A PALMITATE, VITAMIN D3), CREAM CHEESE (PASTEURIZED MILK AND CREAM, WHEY PROTEIN CONCENTRATE, SALT, CAROB BEAN GUM, XANTHAN GUM, CHEESE CULTURE), WHITE BREAD (ENRICHED WHEAT FLOUR (FLOUR, MALTED BARLEY FLOUR, NIACIN, IRON (FERROUS SULFATE, REDUCED IRON), THIAMINE MONONITRATE, RIBOFLAVIN, FOLIC ACID), WATER, YEAST, SALT, SOYBEAN OIL, SUGAR, MALT, DOUGH CONDITIONERS (ASCORBIC ACID, CALCIUM SULFATE, SODIUM STEAROYL LACTYLATE), CALCIUM PROPIONATE (PRESERVATIVE)), CHEDDAR (MILK, CULTURES, SALT, ENZYMES, ANNATTO (COLOR)), BUTTER (CREAM, NATURAL FLAVOR), ENRICHED UNBLEACHED FLOUR (WHEAT FLOUR, MALTED BARLEY FLOUR, NIACIN, IRON, THIAMINE, RIBOFLAVIN, FOLIC ACID), MUSTARD (WATER, VINEGAR, MUSTARD SEED, SALT, WHITE WINE, FRUIT PECTIN, CITRIC ACID, TARTARIC ACID, SUGAR, SPICE), PARSLEY, BLACK PEPPER

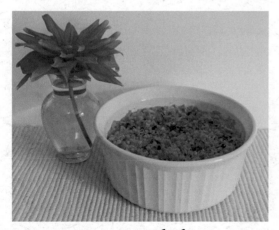

Macaroni and Cheese

Manicotti

Serves 6

Preheat oven to 350°F

6 large manicotti shells

2 cups shredded mozzarella cheese, divided
1 cup ricotta cheese
3 Tbsp chopped fresh basil
12 oz low sodium pasta sauce
1/4 cup fresh grated Parmesan cheese

Spray an 8 x 8 glass baking dish with cooking spray. Cook pasta as per package directions. Drain, rinse with cool water and dry on paper towels. In a medium bowl, stir together 1 1/2 cups mozzarella with ricotta and fresh basil. Stuff into pasta using a teaspoon. Spoon 1/3 of pasta sauce into bottom of glass baking dish. Arrange stuffed pasta over sauce. Pour remaining sauce over pasta. Sprinkle with remaining mozzarella cheese. Bake for 15 minutes. Sprinkle with Parmesan and bake for another 10 minutes. Serve immediately.

Manicotti

Nutrition Facts	
6 servings per container	
Serving size	**(154g)**

Amount Per Serving	
Calories	**310**

	% Daily Value*
Total Fat 17g	22%
Saturated Fat 10g	50%
Trans Fat 0g	
Cholesterol 55mg	18%
Sodium 300mg	13%
Total Carbohydrate 21g	8%
Dietary Fiber 1g	4%
Total Sugars 4g	
Includes 0g Added Sugars	0%
Protein 19g	
Vitamin D 0.1mcg	0%
Calcium 430mg	35%
Iron 1.3mg	8%
Potassium 230mg	4%

* The % Daily Value (DV) tells you how much a nutrient in a serving of food contributes to a daily diet. 2,000 calories a day is used for general nutrition advice.

INGREDIENTS: MARINARA SAUCE (TOMATO PUREE (WATER, TOMATO PASTE), DICED TOMATOES IN TOMATO JUICE, CANOLA OIL, CONTAINS LESS THAN 1% OF: SALT, DEHYDRATED ONIONS, DEHYDRATED GARLIC, SPICES, CITRIC ACID), RICOTTA (MILK PASTEURIZED, MILK NONFAT, VINEGAR, MILK FAT, GUAR GUM, CARRAGEENAN, XANTHAN GUM), CHEDDAR (MILK, CULTURES, SALT, ENZYMES, ANNATTO (COLOR)), DURUM WHEAT SEMOLINA, NIACIN, FERROUS SULFATE, THIAMINE MONONITRATE, RIBOFLAVIN, FOLIC ACID., CHEESE, PARMESAN, LOW SODIUM, BASIL

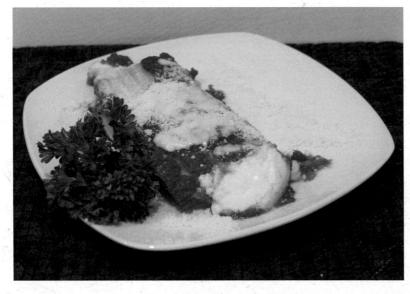

Manicotti

Moon Chilli

This recipe is from my neighbour. Best chilli ever.

Serves 12

1 lb lean ground beef
1 lb ground pork
2 stalks chopped celery
1 small package frozen mixed vegetables
corn niblets (optional)
1 can no salt added red kidney beans, undrained
1 can no salt added white kidney beans, undrained
1 can no salt added seasoned stewed tomatoes, undrained
1 can no salt added seasoned chilli stewed tomatoes, undrained (if unavailable, you can use Italian tomatoes and add chilli powder)
1 package no sodium Mrs. Dash™. chilli seasoning

In a Dutch oven on the stove, sauté onion, ground beef and pork together until cooked. Add celery, vegetables and pepper to taste. Add kidney beans (do not drain). Simmer until celery is still crunchy. Add tomatoes and Mrs. Dash™. Do not overcook. You can eat it now but is better if kept in refrigerator overnight and reheated next day.

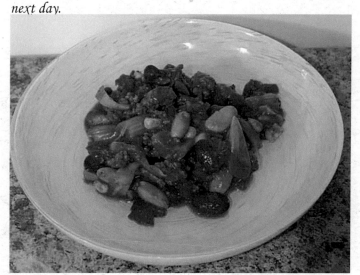

Moon Chilli

Moon Chili

Nutrition Facts		
12 servings per container		
Serving size		**(279g)**
Amount Per Serving		
Calories		**290**
		% Daily Value*
Total Fat 8g		10%
Saturated Fat 3g		15%
Trans Fat 0g		
Cholesterol 50mg		17%
Sodium 70mg		3%
Total Carbohydrate 31g		11%
Dietary Fiber 8g		29%
Total Sugars 3g		
Includes 0g Added Sugars		0%
Protein 25g		
Vitamin D 0.1mcg		0%
Calcium 80mg		6%
Iron 4.6mg		25%
Potassium 690mg		15%

* The % Daily Value (DV) tells you how much a nutrient in a serving of food contributes to a daily diet. 2,000 calories a day is used for general nutrition advice.

INGREDIENTS: TOMATOES, TOMATO JUICE, CITRIC ACID, CALCIUM CHLORIDE., BEANS, KIDNEY, RED, MATURE SEEDS, COOKED, BOILED, WITHOUT SALT, BEANS, KIDNEY, ALL TYPES, MATURE SEEDS, COOKED, BOILED, WITHOUT SALT, GROUND BEEF, PORK, GROUND, 96% LEAN / 4% FAT, RAW, MIXED VEGETABLES (PEAS, CARROTS, GREEN BEANS, CORN), CORN, SWEET, YELLOW, FROZEN, KERNELS CUT OFF COB, BOILED, DRAINED, WITHOUT SALT, CELERY, CHILI PEPPER, WHEAT FLOUR, CORN STARCH, DRIED ONION, CUMIN, SUGAR, GARLIC POWDER, ONION POWDER, RED PEPPER, CITRIC ACID, OREGANO.

Pancake Batter

My son used to like to roll these pancakes up, sprinkle with lemon juice and sugar and eat them. They are also good as dessert pancakes rolled up and drizzled with a fruit sauce, garnished with whipping cream or sprinkled with confectioner's sugar.

Serves 3

1 cup all purpose flour

1 egg

Dash salt (less than an 1/8 tsp)

2 Tbsp oil

1 cup milk mixed with 2 Tbsp water

Sift flour and salt in a mixing bowl. Make a well in centre. Drop in egg and oil. Stir rapidly until well blended. Add milk a little at a time, stirring continuously. Cook in hot oil and serve with butter and syrup.

Pancake Batter

Nutrition Facts	
Serving Size: (159g)	
Servings Per Container: 3	

Amount Per Serving	
Calories 300	Calories from Fat 120

	% Daily Value*
Total Fat 13g	**20%**
Saturated Fat 2g	**10%**
Trans Fat 0g	
Cholesterol 70mg	**23%**
Sodium 115mg	**5%**
Total Carbohydrate 36g	**12%**
Dietary Fiber 1g	**4%**
Sugars 4g	
Protein 9g	

Vitamin A 4%	•	Vitamin C 0%
Calcium 10%	•	Iron 10%

* Percent Daily Values are based on a 2,000 calorie diet. Your daily values may be higher or lower depending on your calorie needs:

	Calories:	2,000	2,500
Total Fat	Less than	65g	80g
Sat Fat	Less than	20g	25g
Cholesterol	Less than	300mg	300mg
Sodium	Less than	2,400mg	2,400mg
Total Carbohydrate		300g	375g
Dietary Fiber		25g	30g

INGREDIENTS: MILK (PASTEURIZED REDUCED FAT MILK, VITAMIN A PALMITATE, VITAMIN D3), ENRICHED UNBLEACHED FLOUR (WHEAT FLOUR, MALTED BARLEY FLOUR, NIACIN, IRON, THIAMINE, RIBOFLAVIN, FOLIC ACID), EGG, WATER, OIL, VEGETABLE, NATREON CANOLA, HIGH STABILITY, NON TRANS, HIGH OLEIC (70%), SALT

Pasta Sauce

Try different tomatoes or combinations of tomatoes until you find a blend you like best.

Serves 4

Preheat oven to 350°F

8 Roma tomatoes

1 pint grape tomatoes

(You can use any variety of tomatoes you choose for different flavours and grape tomatoes are optional)

Olive oil

1/2 cup diced onions

2 cloves garlic minced

2 cans 1% sodium tomato paste

Fresh basil to taste

Italian seasoning to taste

Place a large piece of tin foil on a baking pan. Halve tomatoes and place on foil cut side up. Sprinkle with onions and garlic. Drizzle with olive oil. Fold foil and close into a packet. Bake for 45-60 minutes until done. Cool. Puree in a food processor or blender. In a large pot, cook with spices until ready to serve.

Pasta Sauce

Nutrition Facts

Serving Size: (329g)
Servings Per Container: 4

Amount Per Serving	
Calories 250	Calories from Fat 130

	% Daily Value*
Total Fat 15g	23%
Saturated Fat 2g	10%
Trans Fat 0g	
Cholesterol 0mg	0%
Sodium 65mg	3%
Total Carbohydrate 28g	9%
Dietary Fiber 7g	28%
Sugars 16g	
Protein 6g	

Vitamin A 60%	•	Vitamin C 100%	
Calcium 6%	•	Iron 20%	

* Percent Daily Values are based on a 2,000 calorie diet. Your daily values may be higher or lower depending on your calorie needs:

	Calories:	2,000	2,500
Total Fat	Less than	65g	80g
Sat Fat	Less than	20g	25g
Cholesterol	Less than	300mg	300mg
Sodium	Less than	2,400mg	2,400mg
Total Carbohydrate		300g	375g
Dietary Fiber		25g	30g

INGREDIENTS: GRAPE TOMATOES, TOMATOES, TOMATO PASTE (TOMATOES, SPICES, NATURAL FLAVORS, CITRIC ACID), ONIONS, OLIVE OIL, GARLIC, BASIL, FENNEL, OREGANO

Potatoes Romanoff

Serves 10

Preheat oven to 350°F

6 large potatoes
1 large container sour cream
1 1/2 cups shredded sharp cheddar, divided
1 bunch chopped green onions
pepper
paprika

Bake potatoes in skins until fork tender. Peel skins and shred potatoes into a large bowl. Stir in sour cream, 1 cup of the cheese, onion, and pepper to taste. Scoop into 2-quart buttered casserole dish. Top with remaining cheese and sprinkle with paprika. Cover and refrigerate several hours or overnight. Bake uncovered for 30-40 minutes.

Potatoes Romanoff

Nutrition Facts

Serving Size: (296g)
Servings Per Container: 10

Amount Per Serving

Calories 290 | Calories from Fat 90

	% Daily Value*
Total Fat 10g	**15%**
Saturated Fat 6g	**30%**
Trans Fat 0g	
Cholesterol 35mg	**12%**
Sodium 190mg	**8%**
Total Carbohydrate 40g	**13%**
Dietary Fiber 6g	**24%**
Sugars 3g	
Protein 10g	

Vitamin A 10%	•	Vitamin C 40%
Calcium 20%	•	Iron 8%

* Percent Daily Values are based on a 2,000 calorie diet. Your daily values may be higher or lower depending on your calorie needs:

	Calories:	2,000	2,500
Total Fat	Less than	65g	80g
Sat Fat	Less than	20g	25g
Cholesterol	Less than	300mg	300mg
Sodium	Less than	2,400mg	2,400mg
Total Carbohydrate		300g	375g
Dietary Fiber		25g	30g

INGREDIENTS: POTATOES, SOUR CREAM (CULTURED CREAM, SKIM MILK, VITAMIN A PALMITATE), CHEDDAR (MILK, CULTURES, SALT, ENZYMES, ANNATTO (COLOR)), GREEN ONION, PAPRIKA, BLACK PEPPER

Scalloped Potatoes

Serves 8

Preheat oven to 350°F

4-5 large potatoes peeled and sliced

1/2 onion diced

3 Tbsp unsalted butter

3 Tbsp flour

1/2 tsp pepper

1/4 tsp cayenne pepper

1/4 tsp garlic powder

2 cups milk

1 1/2 cups shredded sharp cheddar

Butter baking dish. Melt butter in saucepan. Mix in flour and cook on medium heat until bubbly. Add peppers, garlic powder and milk. Stir and cook until thickened and almost a boil. Remove from heat and stir in cheese. Layer half of potatoes in baking dish. Top with half of onions. Pour half of sauce mixture over potatoes and onions, layer remaining potatoes and onions and cover with rest of sauce. Cover and bake for 1 hour. Uncover and continue to bake for 30 more minutes.

Scalloped Potatoes

Nutrition Facts

Serving Size: (314g)
Servings Per Container: 8

Amount Per Serving

Calories 260   Calories from Fat 60

	% Daily Value*
Total Fat 7g	**11%**
Saturated Fat 4g	**20%**
Trans Fat 0g	
Cholesterol 20mg	**7%**
Sodium 90mg	**4%**
Total Carbohydrate 43g	**14%**
Dietary Fiber 6g	**24%**
Sugars 6g	
Protein 7g	

Vitamin A 6%	•	Vitamin C 35%
Calcium 10%	•	Iron 8%

* Percent Daily Values are based on a 2,000 calorie diet. Your daily values may be higher or lower depending on your calorie needs:

		Calories:	2,000	2,500
Total Fat	Less than		65g	80g
Sat Fat	Less than		20g	25g
Cholesterol	Less than		300mg	300mg
Sodium	Less than		2,400mg	2,400mg
Total Carbohydrate			300g	375g
Dietary Fiber			25g	30g

INGREDIENTS: POTATOES, MILK (PASTEURIZED REDUCED FAT MILK, VITAMIN A PALMITATE, VITAMIN D3), ONIONS, BUTTER (CREAM, NATURAL FLAVOR), CHEDDAR (MILK, CULTURES, SALT, ENZYMES, ANNATTO (COLOR)), ENRICHED UNBLEACHED FLOUR (WHEAT FLOUR, MALTED BARLEY FLOUR, NIACIN, IRON, THIAMINE, RIBOFLAVIN, FOLIC ACID), BLACK PEPPER, GARLIC POWDER, CAYENNE PEPPER

Sunshine Jam

My children loved this jam. They said it was like a mouthful of sunshine. It only turns out really well on a year when peaches and apricots are ripened nicely. Sadly, not every year is that so.

Serves 10

1 1/2 cups finely chopped peeled peaches

1 1/4 cups finely chopped unpeeled apricots

6 1/2 cups sugar

1/3 cup lemon juice

2 pouches liquid pectin

Mix peaches, apricots and sugar. Mix well. Let stand for 10 minutes. Stir in 2 pouches of liquid pectin and 1/3 cup of lemon juice. Stir for three minutes until most of the sugar is dissolved. Pour into clean jars or plastic containers. Cover and let stand at room temperature until set. (may take up to 24 hours). Store in freezer. Keeps in refrigerator for 3 weeks.

Sunshine Jam

Nutrition Facts

Serving Size: (0.0g)
Servings Per Container: 10

Amount Per Serving

Calories 80   Calories from Fat 0

% Daily Value*

Total Fat 0g	**0%**
Saturated Fat 0g	**0%**
Trans Fat 0g	
Cholesterol 0mg	**0%**
Sodium 0mg	**0%**
Total Carbohydrate 19g	**6%**
Dietary Fiber 0g	**0%**
Sugars 19g	
Protein 0g	

Vitamin A 2%	•		Vitamin C 2%
Calcium 0%	•		Iron 0%

* Percent Daily Values are based on a 2,000 calorie diet. Your daily values may be higher or lower depending on your calorie needs:

		Calories:	2,000	2,500
Total Fat	Less than		65g	80g
Sat Fat	Less than		20g	25g
Cholesterol	Less than		300mg	300mg
Sodium	Less than		2,400mg	2,400mg
Total Carbohydrate			300g	375g
Dietary Fiber			25g	30g

INGREDIENTS: SUGAR, PEACHES, APRICOTS, PECTIN, LEMON JUICE

PORK

To avoid gravies with pork, I use fruit. Apples and apricots and pineapple work very well and are sodium free.

1. Pork Chops

2. Pork Chops and Rice

3. Spiced Apple Pork Roast

4. Apricot Pork Roast

Pork Chops

Serves 2

1 apple, peeled, cored and sliced into wedges
2 pork chops
1 Tbsp butter
1 Tbsp vegetable oil

Melt butter in a frying pan. Add oil and mix. Add apple slices and pork chops. Sauté until pork chops are cooked and apple slices are browned. The combination of oil and butter gives an excellent flavour to the pork.

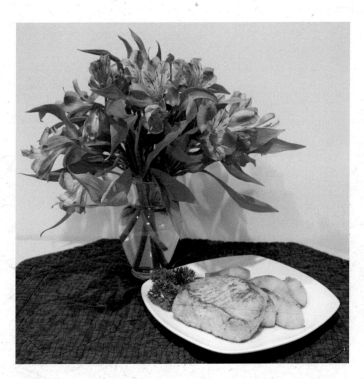

Pork Chops

Nutrition Facts	
Serving Size: (210g)	
Servings Per Container: 2	

Amount Per Serving

Calories 300	Calories from Fat 170

	% Daily Value*
Total Fat 19g	**29%**
Saturated Fat 6g	**30%**
Trans Fat 0g	
Cholesterol 65mg	**22%**
Sodium 85mg	**4%**
Total Carbohydrate 14g	**5%**
Dietary Fiber 1g	**4%**
Sugars 11g	
Protein 20g	

Vitamin A 4%	•	Vitamin C 8%
Calcium 2%	•	Iron 4%

* Percent Daily Values are based on a 2,000 calorie diet. Your daily values may be higher or lower depending on your calorie needs:

	Calories:	2,000	2,500
Total Fat	Less than	65g	80g
Sat Fat	Less than	20g	25g
Cholesterol	Less than	300mg	300mg
Sodium	Less than	2,400mg	2,400mg
Total Carbohydrate		300g	375g
Dietary Fiber		25g	30g

INGREDIENTS: APPLES, PORK, FRESH, LOIN, CENTER RIB (CHOPS OR ROASTS), BONELESS, SEPARABLE LEAN ONLY, RAW, BUTTER (CREAM, SALT), OIL, VEGETABLE, NATREON CANOLA, HIGH STABILITY, NON TRANS, HIGH OLEIC (70%)

Pork Chops and Rice

Serves 2

Preheat oven to 350°F

2 pork chops

1 Tbsp cooking oil

1 can no salt added cream of mushroom soup

3/4 cup milk

3/4 cup uncooked instant white rice

1/8 tsp onion powder

1/8 tsp garlic powder

Pepper

In a skillet, brown pork chops in oil over medium heat. Set aside. In an ungreased 8 x 8 glass baking dish, combine soup, milk, rice and seasonings. Mix well. Top with pork chops. Cover and bake for 45 minutes. Uncover and bake for 5 more minutes. Let stand for 10 minutes and serve.

Pork Chops and Rice

Nutrition Facts

Serving Size: (434g)
Servings Per Container: 2

Amount Per Serving

Calories 670   Calories from Fat 250

	% Daily Value*
Total Fat 28g	**43%**
Saturated Fat 6g	**30%**
Trans Fat 0g	
Cholesterol 65mg	**22%**
Sodium 115mg	**5%**
Total Carbohydrate 72g	**24%**
Dietary Fiber 1g	**4%**
Sugars 6g	
Protein 30g	

Vitamin A 4%	•	Vitamin C 0%
Calcium 15%	•	Iron 25%

* Percent Daily Values are based on a 2,000 calorie diet. Your daily values may be higher or lower depending on your calorie needs:

	Calories:	2,000	2,500
Total Fat	Less than	65g	80g
Sat Fat	Less than	20g	25g
Cholesterol	Less than	300mg	300mg
Sodium	Less than	2,400mg	2,400mg
Total Carbohydrate		300g	375g
Dietary Fiber		25g	30g

INGREDIENTS: WATER, MUSHROOMS, VEGETABLE OIL, MODIFIED CORN STARCH, WHEAT FLOUR, CREAM (MILK), WHEY POWDER, SOY PROTEIN ISOLATE, TOMATO PASTE, SPICE EXTRACT, YEAST EXTRACT, DEHYDRATED GARLIC FLAVOUR, MILK (PASTEURIZED REDUCED FAT MILK, VITAMIN A PALMITATE, VITAMIN D3), PORK, FRESH, LOIN, CENTER RIB (CHOPS OR ROASTS), BONELESS, SEPARABLE LEAN ONLY, RAW, RICE, WHITE, LONG-GRAIN, REGULAR, RAW, ENRICHED, OIL, VEGETABLE, NATREON CANOLA, HIGH STABILITY, NON TRANS, HIGH OLEIC (70%), GARLIC POWDER, ONION POWDER, BLACK PEPPER

Spiced Apple Pork Roast

Serves 10

Preheat oven to 325°F

Rub

1 tsp ground ginger
½ tsp ground nutmeg
½ tsp ground cinnamon

4-5 lb pork loin centre cut roast

Sauce Ingredients

2 medium apples, peeled, cored and cut into wedges
1/4 cup honey
1/4 cup water
1 Tbsp lemon juice
1/4 tsp ground ginger
1/4 tsp ground nutmeg
1/4 tsp ground cinnamon

Combine rub ingredients and rub onto outside of pork roast. Place meat fat side up on rack in shallow roasting pan. Roast uncovered until meat is cooked. Let stand 15 minutes.

For sauce, combine remaining ingredients (except apple slices) and bring to a boil. Add apples, cover and simmer for 8-10 minutes until apples are just tender. Serve with meat.

Spiced Apple Pork Roast

Nutrition Facts

Serving Size: (230g)
Servings Per Container: 10

Amount Per Serving

Calories 320   Calories from Fat 110

% Daily Value*

Total Fat 12g	**18%**
Saturated Fat 4g	**20%**
Trans Fat 0g	
Cholesterol 100mg	**33%**
Sodium 80mg	**3%**
Total Carbohydrate 12g	**4%**
Dietary Fiber <1g	**3%**
Sugars 10g	
Protein 40g	

Vitamin A 0%	•	Vitamin C 4%
Calcium 2%	•	Iron 8%

* Percent Daily Values are based on a 2,000 calorie diet. Your daily values may be higher or lower depending on your calorie needs:

	Calories:	2,000	2,500
Total Fat	Less than	65g	80g
Sat Fat	Less than	20g	25g
Cholesterol	Less than	300mg	300mg
Sodium	Less than	2,400mg	2,400mg
Total Carbohydrate		300g	375g
Dietary Fiber		25g	30g

INGREDIENTS: PORK, FRESH, LOIN, CENTER RIB (CHOPS OR ROASTS), BONELESS, SEPARABLE LEAN ONLY, RAW, APPLES, HONEY, WATER, LEMON JUICE, GROUND GINGER, CINNAMON, NUTMEG

Apricot Pork Roast

Serves 10

Preheat oven to 350°F

1 pork loin roast (4 lb)
1 jar apple jelly (10 oz)
1 cup apple juice
3/4 cup fresh apricots or dried apricots chopped
1/2 tsp cardamom
1 Tbsp cornstarch
2 Tbsp water

Bake roast uncovered in a small roasting pan for 1 1/2 hours. Combine juice, jelly and cardamom in a saucepan. Cook over medium heat until heated through. Brush some sauce over roast and continue baking for another 40-60 minutes until well cooked. Place roast on a serving platter.

Pour roast pan drippings into saucepan with remaining sauce. Add apricots and cook over medium heat until dried apricots are softened or fresh are cooked (3-5 minutes). Do not overcook fresh apricots or they will be mushy. Combine cornstarch and water until smooth. Add to apricot mixture and bring to a boil. Cook for a couple of minutes until thickened. Serve over roast.

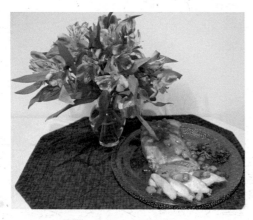

Apricot Pork Roast

Apricot Pork Roast

Nutrition Facts

Serving Size: (255g)
Servings Per Container: 10

Amount Per Serving

Calories 400	Calories from Fat 110

	% Daily Value*
Total Fat 12g	**18%**
Saturated Fat 4g	**20%**
Trans Fat 0g	
Cholesterol 100mg	**33%**
Sodium 85mg	**4%**
Total Carbohydrate 32g	**11%**
Dietary Fiber <1g	**4%**
Sugars 28g	
Protein 40g	

Vitamin A 10%	•	Vitamin C 2%
Calcium 2%	•	Iron 10%

* Percent Daily Values are based on a 2,000 calorie diet. Your daily values may be higher or lower depending on your calorie needs:

	Calories:	2,000	2,500
Total Fat	Less than	65g	80g
Sat Fat	Less than	20g	25g
Cholesterol	Less than	300mg	300mg
Sodium	Less than	2,400mg	2,400mg
Total Carbohydrate		300g	375g
Dietary Fiber		25g	30g

INGREDIENTS: PORK, FRESH, LOIN, CENTER RIB (CHOPS OR ROASTS), BONELESS, SEPARABLE LEAN ONLY, RAW, APPLE JUICE (HIGH FRUCTOSE CORN SYRUP, CITRIC ACID, FRUIT PECTIN, CORN SYRUP,, APPLE JUICE (APPLE JUICE, WATER, APPLE JUICE CONCENTRATE), DRIED APRICOTS (DRIED APRICOTS, SULFUR DIOXIDE (FOR COLOR RETENTION), POTASSIUM SORBATE (PRESERVATIVE)), WATER, CORNSTARCH, CARDAMOM

VEGETABLES

1. Asparagus with Zesty Hollandaise Sauce

2. Broccoli Casserole

3. Beets

4. Caramelized Ginger Carrots

5. Green Beans

6. Carrots and Asparagus

7. Stuffed Green Peppers

8. Vegetable Fettuccine

9. Vegetable Casserole

Asparagus with Zesty Hollandaise Sauce

Serves 4

1 lb asparagus

Sauce

1/4 cup unsalted butter, softened
2 egg yolks
1/4 tsp grated orange peel (zest)
1 tsp orange juice
1/4 cup sour cream

Melt butter in saucepan and cool.

Trim ends off of asparagus. Simmer in water in a skillet until cooked but crunchy. Drain.

While asparagus is cooking, add egg yolks to cooled butter, cook and stir until it thickens. Remove from heat and stir in orange peel and juice. Return to heat and cook until thickened, 2-3 minutes, stirring constantly. Remove from heat. Blend sour cream into hot mixture and serve over asparagus.

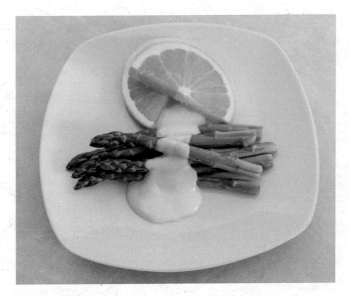

Asparagus with Zesty Hollandaise Sauce

Asparagus with Zesty Hollandaise Sauce

Nutrition Facts

Serving Size: (31g)
Servings Per Container: 4

Amount Per Serving

Calories 150	Calories from Fat 130

	% Daily Value*
Total Fat 15g	23%
Saturated Fat 9g	45%
Trans Fat 0g	
Cholesterol 130mg	43%
Sodium 15mg	1%
Total Carbohydrate 1g	0%
Dietary Fiber 0g	0%
Sugars 0g	
Protein 2g	

Vitamin A 10%	•	Vitamin C 2%
Calcium 4%	•	Iron 2%

* Percent Daily Values are based on a 2,000 calorie diet. Your daily values may be higher or lower depending on your calorie needs:

	Calories:	2,000	2,500
Total Fat	Less than	65g	80g
Sat Fat	Less than	20g	25g
Cholesterol	Less than	300mg	300mg
Sodium	Less than	2,400mg	2,400mg
Total Carbohydrate		300g	375g
Dietary Fiber		25g	30g

INGREDIENTS: BUTTER (CREAM, NATURAL FLAVOR), SOUR CREAM (CULTURED CREAM, SKIM MILK, VITAMIN A PALMITATE), EGG YOLK, ORANGE JUICE, ORANGE ZEST

Broccoli Casserole

Serves 6

Preheat oven to 350°F

1 lb broccoli

2 onions, peeled and diced coarsely

1/8 cup unsalted butter, melted

2 Tbsp flour

1 cup milk

1 (3 oz) package cream cheese, softened

1/2 cup shredded cheddar cheese

Topping

1 cup fresh bread crumbs

1/8 cup melted unsalted butter

Steam broccoli and onions until tender but crunchy. Place in a casserole dish.

Melt butter in a sauce pan and whisk in flour. Add milk. Cook over medium heat, stirring constantly, until thickened and bubbly. Reduce heat, add cream cheese and cook until smooth.

Pour sauce mixture over vegetables, tossing lightly. Sprinkle cheese over top.

Mix bread crumbs and melted butter and sprinkle over top.

Bake 40-45 minutes until heated through.

Broccoli Casserole

Nutrition Facts

Serving Size: (233g)
Servings Per Container: 6

Amount Per Serving

Calories 450 | Calories from Fat 230

	% Daily Value*
Total Fat 25g	**38%**
Saturated Fat 15g	**75%**
Trans Fat 0g	
Cholesterol 70mg	**23%**
Sodium 340mg	**14%**
Total Carbohydrate 44g	**15%**
Dietary Fiber 4g	**16%**
Sugars 7g	
Protein 12g	

Vitamin A 25%	•	Vitamin C 120%
Calcium 25%	•	Iron 15%

* Percent Daily Values are based on a 2,000 calorie diet. Your daily values may be higher or lower depending on your calorie needs:

	Calories:	2,000	2,500
Total Fat	Less than	65g	80g
Sat Fat	Less than	20g	25g
Cholesterol	Less than	300mg	300mg
Sodium	Less than	2,400mg	2,400mg
Total Carbohydrate		300g	375g
Dietary Fiber		25g	30g

INGREDIENTS: BROCCOLI, MILK (PASTEURIZED REDUCED FAT MILK, VITAMIN A PALMITATE, VITAMIN D3), WHITE BREAD (ENRICHED WHEAT FLOUR (FLOUR, MALTED BARLEY FLOUR, NIACIN, IRON (FERROUS SULFATE, REDUCED IRON), THIAMINE MONONITRATE, RIBOFLAVIN, FOLIC ACID), WATER, YEAST, SALT, SOYBEAN OIL, SUGAR, MALT, DOUGH CONDITIONERS (ASCORBIC ACID, CALCIUM SULFATE, SODIUM STEAROYL LACTYLATE), CALCIUM PROPIONATE (PRESERVATIVE)), ONIONS, BUTTER (CREAM, NATURAL FLAVOR), ENRICHED UNBLEACHED FLOUR (WHEAT FLOUR, MALTED BARLEY FLOUR, NIACIN, IRON, THIAMINE, RIBOFLAVIN, FOLIC ACID), CREAM CHEESE (MILK, CHEESE CULTURES, SALT, GUAR GUM), CHEDDAR (MILK, CULTURES, SALT, ENZYMES, ANNATTO (COLOR))

Beets

When growing up we always boiled beets. Baking them this way, they are sweeter and more flavourful.

Serves 4

2 cups peeled, sliced beets
2 tsp butter

Cut off ends of raw beets and peel like potatoes. Slice beets. Spread butter in the centre of a piece of tin foil. Place sliced beets on tin foil and fold into packet. Bake in oven at 350° F or barbeque until cooked, approximately 20-30 minutes depending on number of beets.

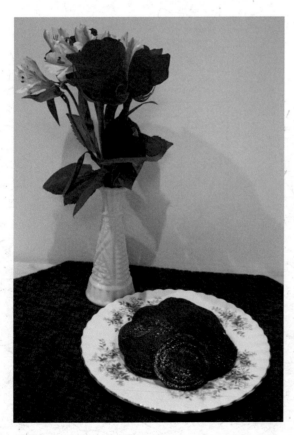

Beets

Beets

Nutrition Facts	
Serving Size: (70g)	
Servings Per Container: 4	

Amount Per Serving	
Calories 45	Calories from Fat 20

	% Daily Value*
Total Fat 2g	**3**%
Saturated Fat 1g	**5**%
Trans Fat 0g	
Cholesterol 5mg	**2**%
Sodium 70mg	**3**%
Total Carbohydrate 7g	**2**%
Dietary Fiber 2g	**8**%
Sugars 5g	
Protein 1g	

Vitamin A 2%	•	Vitamin C 6%
Calcium 2%	•	Iron 4%

* Percent Daily Values are based on a 2,000 calorie diet. Your daily values may be higher or lower depending on your calorie needs:

	Calories:	2,000	2,500
Total Fat	Less than	65g	80g
Sat Fat	Less than	20g	25g
Cholesterol	Less than	300mg	300mg
Sodium	Less than	2,400mg	2,400mg
Total Carbohydrate		300g	375g
Dietary Fiber		25g	30g

INGREDIENTS: BEETS, BUTTER (CREAM, SALT)

Caramelized Ginger Carrots

Serves 4

You can add parsnips, increasing butter, sugar and ginger for a change. You may need more butter, sugar and ginger depending on the number and size of vegetables.

3 medium carrots
1 Tbsp butter
1 Tbsp brown sugar
1/2 tsp ground ginger

Peel and cut ends off of carrots. Cut into 3-inch pieces (slice and quarter larger pieces).

Simmer carrots in water in a skillet until cooked but crunchy. Drain. Add butter, sugar and ginger. Toss to coat and continue to cook until caramelized.

Caramelized Ginger Carrots

Nutrition Facts

Serving Size: (23g)
Servings Per Container: 4

Amount Per Serving

Calories 45	Calories from Fat 25

% Daily Value*

Total Fat 3g	**5%**
Saturated Fat 2g	**10%**
Trans Fat 0g	
Cholesterol 10mg	**3%**
Sodium 35mg	**1%**
Total Carbohydrate 5g	**2%**
Dietary Fiber 0g	**0%**
Sugars 4g	
Protein 0g	

Vitamin A 50%	•		Vitamin C 2%
Calcium 0%	•		Iron 0%

* Percent Daily Values are based on a 2,000 calorie diet. Your daily values may be higher or lower depending on your calorie needs:

	Calories:	2,000	2,500
Total Fat	Less than	65g	80g
Sat Fat	Less than	20g	25g
Cholesterol	Less than	300mg	300mg
Sodium	Less than	2,400mg	2,400mg
Total Carbohydrate		300g	375g
Dietary Fiber		25g	30g

INGREDIENTS: CARROTS, BUTTER (CREAM, SALT), BROWN SUGAR, GROUND GINGER

Green Beans

Serves 4

1 cup green beans cut approximately 1 1/2 inch length

1 tsp low sodium soy sauce

1/4 tsp sugar

1 tsp sesame seeds

Simmer green beans in water until tender but crunchy. In a bowl, mix remaining ingredients. Add beans and toss. Serve

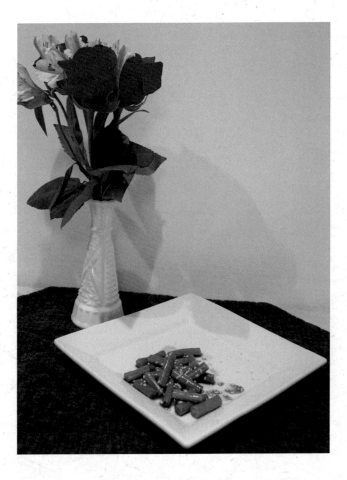

Green Beans

Nutrition Facts

Serving Size: 0.00 (27g)
Servings Per Container: 4

Amount Per Serving

Calories 15	Calories from Fat 0

	% Daily Value*
Total Fat 0g	**0**%
Saturated Fat 0g	**0**%
Trans Fat 0g	
Cholesterol 0mg	**0**%
Sodium 45mg	**2**%
Total Carbohydrate 2g	**1**%
Dietary Fiber <1g	**3**%
Sugars 1g	
Protein 1g	

Vitamin A 4%	•	Vitamin C 6%
Calcium 2%	•	Iron 2%

* Percent Daily Values are based on a 2,000 calorie diet.
Your daily values may be higher or lower depending on
your calorie needs:

	Calories:	2,000	2,500
Total Fat	Less than	65g	80g
Sat Fat	Less than	20g	25g
Cholesterol	Less than	300mg	300mg
Sodium	Less than	2,400mg	2,400mg
Total Carbohydrate		300g	375g
Dietary Fiber		25g	30g

INGREDIENTS: SNAP PEAS, SOY SAUCE, LOW SODIUM- LA CHOY, SESAME SEEDS, SUGAR

Carrots and Asparagus

Serves 4

2 medium carrots

12 asparagus spears

1 Tbsp unsalted butter

2 Tbsp grated Parmesan cheese

Peel and cut carrots. Place in a skillet with water and simmer until tender. Add asparagus and simmer for one more minute. Drain. Add butter, toss and cook for another minute or two. Sprinkle with Parmesan cheese and serve.

Carrots and Asparagus

Nutrition Facts

Serving Size: (85g)
Servings Per Container: 4

Amount Per Serving

Calories 60   Calories from Fat 30

                                          % Daily Value*

Total Fat 3.5g	**5%**
Saturated Fat 2g	**10%**
Trans Fat 0g	
Cholesterol 10mg	**3%**
Sodium 65mg	**3%**
Total Carbohydrate 5g	**2%**
Dietary Fiber 2g	**8%**
Sugars 2g	
Protein 2g	

Vitamin A 110%	•	Vitamin C 8%
Calcium 4%	•	Iron 6%

* Percent Daily Values are based on a 2,000 calorie diet. Your daily values may be higher or lower depending on your calorie needs:

	Calories:	2,000	2,500
Total Fat	Less than	65g	80g
Sat Fat	Less than	20g	25g
Cholesterol	Less than	300mg	300mg
Sodium	Less than	2,400mg	2,400mg
Total Carbohydrate		300g	375g
Dietary Fiber		25g	30g

INGREDIENTS: ASPARAGUS, CARROTS, BUTTER (CREAM, NATURAL FLAVOR), PARMESAN (MILK, CHEESE CULTURES, SALT, ENZYMES)

Stuffed Green Peppers

Serves 2

Preheat oven to 350°F

1 large green pepper

1/4 lb ground beef

2 Tbsp chopped onion

1/2 cup instant white rice

1 cup no salt added tomato sauce, divided

Cut top off green pepper and clean out. Steam until tender but crisp. Prepare rice as per package. Sauté ground beef and onion until cooked. Add rice and 1/3 cup of tomato sauce to beef. Mix well and heat through. Place pepper in a glass baking dish. Fill with beef/rice mixture. Pour remaining tomato sauce over and bake for 1/2 hour.

Stuffed Green Peppers

Nutrition Facts

Serving Size: (322g)
Servings Per Container: 2

Amount Per Serving

Calories 360	Calories from Fat 80

	% Daily Value*
Total Fat 9g	**14%**
Saturated Fat 3.5g	**18%**
Trans Fat 0.5g	
Cholesterol 40mg	**13%**
Sodium 55mg	**2%**
Total Carbohydrate 53g	**18%**
Dietary Fiber 4g	**16%**
Sugars 9g	
Protein 16g	

Vitamin A 20%	•	Vitamin C 140%
Calcium 6%	•	Iron 25%

* Percent Daily Values are based on a 2,000 calorie diet. Your daily values may be higher or lower depending on your calorie needs:

	Calories:	2,000	2,500
Total Fat	Less than	65g	80g
Sat Fat	Less than	20g	25g
Cholesterol	Less than	300mg	300mg
Sodium	Less than	2,400mg	2,400mg
Total Carbohydrate		300g	375g
Dietary Fiber		25g	30g

INGREDIENTS: TOMATO SAUCE, GREEN PEPPERS, GROUND BEEF, RICE, WHITE, LONG-GRAIN, REGULAR, RAW, ENRICHED, ONIONS

Vegetable Fettuccine

Serves 6

4 medium carrots, peeled and sliced diagonally

2 cups broccoli florets

6 oz uncooked fettuccine noodles

3 Tbsp unsalted butter

2 Tbsp all purpose flour

1/2 tsp nutmeg

1 cup milk

1/4 cup fresh grated Parmesan cheese

In a 3-litre saucepan, bring 2 litres of water to a full boil. Add carrots and noodles. Cook over medium heat 6 minutes. Add broccoli. Continue cooking until carrots and broccoli are crisp and tender. Drain and set aside. In same saucepan, melt butter. Stir in flour and nutmeg until smooth and bubbly. Gradually add milk and cook over medium heat until mixture comes to a boil. Boil 1 minute. Stir in noodles and vegetables. Reduce heat and continue cooking until heated through (3-4 minutes). Serve sprinkled with Parmesan cheese.

Vegetable, Fettuccine

Nutrition Facts

Serving Size: (169g)
Servings Per Container: 6

Amount Per Serving

Calories 160   Calories from Fat 80

	% Daily Value*
Total Fat 8g	**12%**
Saturated Fat 5g	**25%**
Trans Fat 0g	
Cholesterol 25mg	**8%**
Sodium 180mg	**8%**
Total Carbohydrate 16g	**5%**
Dietary Fiber 3g	**12%**
Sugars 5g	
Protein 6g	

Vitamin A 150%	•	Vitamin C 50%	
Calcium 10%	•	Iron 8%	

* Percent Daily Values are based on a 2,000 calorie diet. Your daily values may be higher or lower depending on your calorie needs:

	Calories:	2,000	2,500
Total Fat	Less than	65g	80g
Sat Fat	Less than	20g	25g
Cholesterol	Less than	300mg	300mg
Sodium	Less than	2,400mg	2,400mg
Total Carbohydrate		300g	375g
Dietary Fiber		25g	30g

INGREDIENTS: CARROTS, MILK (PASTEURIZED REDUCED FAT MILK, VITAMIN A PALMITATE, VITAMIN D3), BROCCOLI, FETTUCCINE PASTA, BUTTER (CREAM, NATURAL FLAVOR), ENRICHED UNBLEACHED FLOUR (WHEAT FLOUR, MALTED BARLEY FLOUR, NIACIN, IRON, THIAMINE, RIBOFLAVIN, FOLIC ACID), PARMESAN (MILK, CHEESE CULTURES, SALT, ENZYMES), NUTMEG

Vegetable Casserole

Serves 4 as a side dish

Preheat oven to 350°F

3 cups bite-size vegetables (broccoli, cauliflower, carrots, onions, zucchini, mushrooms, green beans)
1 can no salt added mushroom soup
1/2 cup shredded cheddar cheese
Parmesan cheese

Grease a casserole dish. Toss vegetables and soup in a bowl and transfer to casserole dish. Cover with shredded cheddar cheese and sprinkle with Parmesan. Bake for 50 minutes until cooked.

Vegetable Casserole

Nutrition Facts

Serving Size: (1.8g)
Servings Per Container: 4

Amount Per Serving

Calories 150	Calories from Fat 90

	% Daily Value*
Total Fat 10g	**15%**
Saturated Fat 3.5g	**18%**
Trans Fat 0g	
Cholesterol 20mg	**7%**
Sodium 140mg	**6%**
Total Carbohydrate 11g	**4%**
Dietary Fiber 2g	**8%**
Sugars 3g	
Protein 6g	

Vitamin A 110%	•	Vitamin C 60%
Calcium 15%	•	Iron 4%

* Percent Daily Values are based on a 2,000 calorie diet. Your daily values may be higher or lower depending on your calorie needs:

	Calories:	2,000	2,500
Total Fat	Less than	65g	80g
Sat Fat	Less than	20g	25g
Cholesterol	Less than	300mg	300mg
Sodium	Less than	2,400mg	2,400mg
Total Carbohydrate		300g	375g
Dietary Fiber		25g	30g

INGREDIENTS: WATER, MUSHROOMS, VEGETABLE OIL, MODIFIED CORN STARCH, WHEAT FLOUR, CREAM (MILK), WHEY POWDER, SOY PROTEIN ISOLATE, TOMATO PASTE, SPICE EXTRACT, YEAST EXTRACT, DEHYDRATED GARLIC FLAVOUR, CARROTS, CAULIFLOWER, BROCCOLI, CHEDDAR (MILK, CULTURES, SALT, ENZYMES, ANNATTO (COLOR))

DESSERTS

The cakes were a challenge but I believe these are good. I hope you enjoy them too.

Pastry is not one of my finer baking points, so I use a lovely one in a roll that you can find in the dairy section at the local grocery store. There are frozen ones available too.

1. Cranberry Pineapple Frozen Dessert

2. Exquisite Lemon Pie

3. Crème Caramel

4. Sparkling Raspberry Pie

5. Banana Coconut Cream Pie

6. Berry Custard Dessert

7. Thanksgiving Cheesecake

8. Creamy Chocolate Dessert

9. Lemon Pudding Cups

10. Icy Dark Sweet Cherries

11. Orange Chiffon Pie

12. Fresh Strawberry Pie

13. Chocolate Cake

14. Chocolate Brownie Cake

15. Carrot Cake

16. White Cake

17. Banana Cake

Cranberry Pineapple Frozen Dessert

Serves 6 depending on the size of the bowls.

1/4 cup sugar

1 can (8 oz) crushed pineapple, drained

1 cup fresh or frozen cranberries

1/2 cup whipping cream, whipped

Blend sugar, pineapple and cranberries in food processor until cranberries are finely chopped. Let stand in a bowl for 10 minutes. Fold in whipping cream. Spoon into dishes or lined muffin cups. Freeze. Take out of the freezer 15-20 minutes before serving. Garnish with sprigs of mint or cranberries.

Cranberry Pineapple Frozen Dessert

Nutrition Facts	
Serving Size: (76g)	
Servings Per Container: 6	

Amount Per Serving	
Calories 100	Calories from Fat 35

	% Daily Value*
Total Fat 3.5g	**5%**
Saturated Fat 2.5g	**13%**
Trans Fat 0g	
Cholesterol 10mg	**3%**
Sodium 0mg	**0%**
Total Carbohydrate 17g	**6%**
Dietary Fiber <1g	**4%**
Sugars 15g	
Protein 1g	

Vitamin A 4%	•	Vitamin C 10%
Calcium 0%	•	Iron 0%

* Percent Daily Values are based on a 2,000 calorie diet. Your daily values may be higher or lower depending on your calorie needs:

	Calories:	2,000	2,500
Total Fat	Less than	65g	80g
Sat Fat	Less than	20g	25g
Cholesterol	Less than	300mg	300mg
Sodium	Less than	2,400mg	2,400mg
Total Carbohydrate		300g	375g
Dietary Fiber		25g	30g

INGREDIENTS: PINEAPPLE (PINEAPPLE, PINEAPPLE JUICE, CITRIC ACID), CRANBERRIES, HEAVY CREAM (HEAVY CREAM, SKIM MILK, CARRAGEENAN), SUGAR

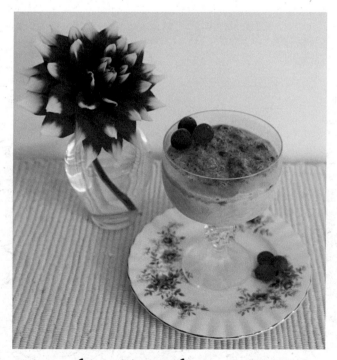

Cranberry Pineapple Frozen Dessert

Exquisite Lemon Pie

Serves 8

Preheat oven to 350°F

1 pie crust

1/2 cup sugar

1/2 cup unsalted butter, melted

1 tsp vanilla

4 large eggs

1 large lemon (use a fresh juicy lemon – makes a difference in outcome)

Wash unpeeled lemon and cut into small pieces, removing seeds. Blend in food processor or blender. Add eggs, butter, vanilla, and sugar until smooth. Place pie crust in pie plate (I use Pillsbury roll out crust found in dairy section). Pour filling into pie plate. Bake for approximately 40-45 minutes until set. Top with whipped cream if desired.

Exquisite Lemon Pie

Nutrition Facts

Serving Size: (78g)
Servings Per Container: 8

Amount Per Serving

Calories 240   Calories from Fat 180

	% Daily Value*
Total Fat 20g	**31**%
Saturated Fat 10g	**50**%
Trans Fat 0g	
Cholesterol 125mg	**42**%
Sodium 170mg	**7**%
Total Carbohydrate 14g	**5**%
Dietary Fiber <1g	**3**%
Sugars 0g	
Protein 3g	

Vitamin A 10%	•	Vitamin C 15%
Calcium 2%	•	Iron 2%

* Percent Daily Values are based on a 2,000 calorie diet. Your daily values may be higher or lower depending on your calorie needs:

	Calories:	2,000	2,500
Total Fat	Less than	65g	80g
Sat Fat	Less than	20g	25g
Cholesterol	Less than	300mg	300mg
Sodium	Less than	2,400mg	2,400mg
Total Carbohydrate		300g	375g
Dietary Fiber		25g	30g

INGREDIENTS: PILLSBURY PIE CRUST, EGG, BUTTER (CREAM, NATURAL FLAVOR), LEMON, VANILLA EXTRACT (WATER, ALCOHOL (35%), SUGAR, VANILLA BEAN EXTRACTIVES)

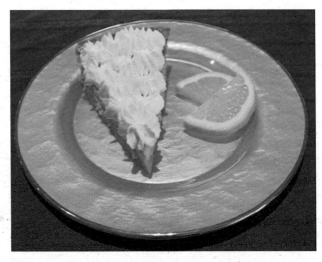

Exquisite Lemon Pie

Crème Caramel

Serves 6

Preheat oven to 325°F and grease six custard cups/ramekins

4 large eggs
2 cups milk
1/2 cup sugar, divided
1 tsp vanilla
1/4 tsp salt

In a small saucepan over medium heat, melt 1/4 cup sugar until it turns a caramel colour, stirring constantly. Pour into greased dishes immediately. With a whisk in a large bowl, beat eggs and remaining 1/4 cup sugar until blended. Add milk, salt and vanilla until well blended. Pour into cups. Place cups in a 9 x 13 glass baking dish. Fill pan with boiling water half way up the sides of the dishes. Bake for 50-55 minutes until toothpick comes out clean.

Place cups in fridge until chilled. When serving, edge cups with a sharp knife, invert onto plate.

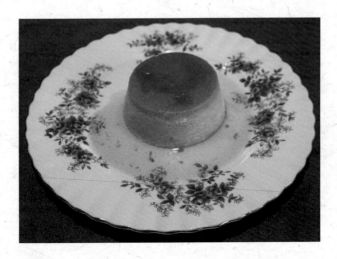

Creme Caramel

Nutrition Facts	
Serving Size: (134g)	
Servings Per Container: 6	

Amount Per Serving	
Calories 170	Calories from Fat 45
	% Daily Value*
Total Fat 5g	**8%**
Saturated Fat 2g	**10%**
Trans Fat 0g	
Cholesterol 130mg	**43%**
Sodium 180mg	**8%**
Total Carbohydrate 23g	**8%**
Dietary Fiber 0g	**0%**
Sugars 23g	
Protein 7g	

Vitamin A 6%	•		Vitamin C 0%
Calcium 10%	•		Iron 4%

* Percent Daily Values are based on a 2,000 calorie diet. Your daily values may be higher or lower depending on your calorie needs:

	Calories:	2,000	2,500
Total Fat	Less than	65g	80g
Sat Fat	Less than	20g	25g
Cholesterol	Less than	300mg	300mg
Sodium	Less than	2,400mg	2,400mg
Total Carbohydrate		300g	375g
Dietary Fiber		25g	30g

INGREDIENTS: MILK (PASTEURIZED REDUCED FAT MILK, VITAMIN A PALMITATE, VITAMIN D3), EGG, SUGAR, VANILLA EXTRACT (WATER, ALCOHOL (35%), SUGAR, VANILLA BEAN EXTRACTIVES), SALT

Sparkling Raspberry Pie

Serves 8

Preheat oven to 375°F

Graham Crust

1 1/3 cups graham cracker crumbs

3 Tbsp sugar

1/4 cup unsalted butter, melted

Place crumbs and sugar in pie plate. Mix well. Pour melted butter in and mix. Press on bottom of pan and up sides. Bake for 8 minutes. Cool.

Filling

1 Tbsp. cornstarch

1/4 cup sugar

1 cup water

1 (3 oz) package raspberry jello

4 cups fresh raspberries

Combine sugar, cornstarch and water in a sauce pan. Bring to a boil. Continue to cook for 2 minutes, stirring constantly. Remove from heat and stir in raspberry jello until dissolved. Cool for approximately 15 minutes. Place raspberries in crust. Pour jello over berries. Chill several hours until set. If desired, garnish with whipped cream.

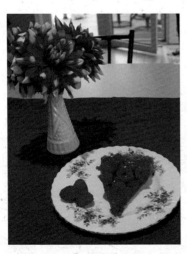

Sparkling Raspberry Pie

Sparkling Raspberry Pie

Nutrition Facts

Serving Size: (139g)
Servings Per Container: 8

Amount Per Serving

Calories 250 — Calories from Fat 70

% Daily Value*

Total Fat 8g	**12%**
Saturated Fat 3.5g	**18%**
Trans Fat 0g	
Cholesterol 15mg	**5%**
Sodium 140mg	**6%**
Total Carbohydrate 44g	**15%**
Dietary Fiber 4g	**16%**
Sugars 28g	
Protein 3g	

Vitamin A 4%	•	Vitamin C 25%	
Calcium 2%	•	Iron 4%	

* Percent Daily Values are based on a 2,000 calorie diet. Your daily values may be higher or lower depending on your calorie needs:

	Calories:	2,000	2,500
Total Fat	Less than	65g	80g
Sat Fat	Less than	20g	25g
Cholesterol	Less than	300mg	300mg
Sodium	Less than	2,400mg	2,400mg
Total Carbohydrate		300g	375g
Dietary Fiber		25g	30g

INGREDIENTS: RASPBERRIES, WATER, GRAHAM CRACKERS (UNBLEACHED ENRICHED FLOUR (WHEAT FLOUR, NIACIN, REDUCED IRON, THIAMINE MONONITRATE {VITAMIN B1}, RIBOFLAVIN {VITAMIN B2}, FOLIC ACID), GRAHAM FLOUR (WHOLE GRAIN WHEAT FLOUR), SUGAR, SOYBEAN OIL, HONEY, LEAVENING (BAKING SODA AND/OR CALCIUM PHOSPHATE), SALT, SOY LECITHIN, ARTIFICIAL FLAVOR), SUGAR, JELL-O RASPBERRY GELATIN, BUTTER (CREAM, NATURAL FLAVOR), CORNSTARCH

Banana Coconut Cream Pie

Serves 10

Preheat oven to 350°F

1/3 cups flaked coconut

2/3 cup quick cooking oats (uncooked)

5 Tbsp unsalted butter

3 cups milk

1/3 cup cornstarch

3 large egg yolks

1/2 cup plus 2 tsp sugar

1 1/2 tsp vanilla

3 large bananas

1/2 cup whipping cream

In a 9 inch pie plate, mix oats, coconut and 3 Tbsp softened butter. Press into pan. Bake for 15 minutes. Cool.

In a saucepan, combine cornstarch, egg yolks, 1/2 cup sugar, milk and remaining 2 Tbsp butter. Cook over medium to low heat, stirring until mixture boils and thickens (approximately one minute). Remove from heat and stir in vanilla.

Slice bananas and layer in cooled crust. Pour custard filling over bananas. Cover with plastic wrap and refrigerate until cold. Whip remaining whipping cream and 2 Tbsp sugar until stiff peaks form and spread over pie.

Banana Coconut Cream Pie

Nutrition Facts

Serving Size: (163g)
Servings Per Container: 10

Amount Per Serving

Calories 290   Calories from Fat 130

	% Daily Value*
Total Fat 14g	**22%**
Saturated Fat 9g	**45%**
Trans Fat 0g	
Cholesterol 85mg	**28%**
Sodium 40mg	**2%**
Total Carbohydrate 35g	**12%**
Dietary Fiber 3g	**12%**
Sugars 21g	
Protein 5g	

Vitamin A 10%	•	Vitamin C 6%
Calcium 10%	•	Iron 2%

* Percent Daily Values are based on a 2,000 calorie diet. Your daily values may be higher or lower depending on your calorie needs.

	Calories:	2,000	2,500
Total Fat	Less than	65g	80g
Sat Fat	Less than	20g	25g
Cholesterol	Less than	300mg	300mg
Sodium	Less than	2,400mg	2,400mg
Total Carbohydrate		300g	375g
Dietary Fiber		25g	30g

INGREDIENTS: MILK (PASTEURIZED REDUCED FAT MILK, VITAMIN A PALMITATE, VITAMIN D3), BANANAS, SUGAR, COCONUT, BUTTER (CREAM, NATURAL FLAVOR), HEAVY CREAM (HEAVY CREAM, SKIM MILK, CARRAGEENAN), OATS, EGG YOLK, CORNSTARCH, VANILLA EXTRACT (WATER, ALCOHOL (35%), SUGAR, VANILLA BEAN EXTRACTIVES)

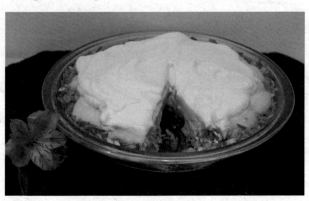

Banana Coconut Cream Pie

Berry Custard Dessert

Very showy for taking to a party.

Serves 10

Preheat oven to 350° F

Pastry

1 cup flour
3/4 cup shredded coconut
6 Tbsp unsalted butter
2 Tbsp sugar
1 large egg yolk

Custard Filling

1 large lemon
6 Tbsp unsalted butter
1/3 cup sugar
1 Tbsp cornstarch
4 large egg yolks
1 cup whipping cream
2 1/2 pints raspberries
1 pint of blueberries
(other fruits can be substituted—cherries, kiwi, grapes, etc.)

Mix coconut pastry ingredients and press into 10-inch tart pan. Prick with a fork and bake until golden (10-15 min.).

Prepare custard filling. Wash lemon and grate 1 tsp of peel and squeeze 2 Tbsp of juice. In a saucepan over low to medium heat, melt butter with sugar and cornstarch until thickened and boils, stirring constantly. Boil 1 minute.

In a small bowl, beat egg yolks with a fork. Stir in a small amount of hot sugar mixture. Slowly add remaining sugar mixture, stirring rapidly. Cook and stir until thickened and coats a spoon (approximately 1 minute).

Remove from heat. Stir in lemon peel and lemon juice. Cover with plastic wrap to prevent a crust forming while cooling in fridge for 1 hour.

In a small bowl, beat whipping cream until stiff peaks form. Fold into custard. Spoon evenly over cooled crust. Arrange berries over custard and refrigerate for approximately 1 hour.

Berry Custard Dessert

Nutrition Facts

Serving Size: (129g)
Servings Per Container: 10

Amount Per Serving

Calories 360 — Calories from Fat 230

	% Daily Value*
Total Fat 25g	**38%**
Saturated Fat 17g	**85%**
Trans Fat 0g	
Cholesterol 70mg	**23%**
Sodium 0mg	**0%**
Total Carbohydrate 31g	**10%**
Dietary Fiber 5g	**20%**
Sugars 14g	
Protein 4g	

Vitamin A 15%	•	Vitamin C 20%
Calcium 2%	•	Iron 6%

* Percent Daily Values are based on a 2,000 calorie diet. Your daily values may be higher or lower depending on your calorie needs:

		Calories	2,000	2,500
Total Fat	Less than		65g	80g
Sat Fat	Less than		20g	25g
Cholesterol	Less than		300mg	300mg
Sodium	Less than		2,400mg	2,400mg
Total Carbohydrate			300g	375g
Dietary Fiber			25g	30g

INGREDIENTS: RASPBERRIES, BLUEBERRIES, COCONUT, BUTTER (CREAM, NATURAL FLAVOR), ENRICHED UNBLEACHED FLOUR (WHEAT FLOUR, MALTED BARLEY FLOUR, NIACIN, IRON, THIAMINE, RIBOFLAVIN, FOLIC ACID), HEAVY CREAM (HEAVY CREAM, SKIM MILK, CARRAGEENAN), SUGAR, EGG YOLK

Berry Custard Dessert"

Thanksgiving Cheesecake

What a fabulous fall flavour this has.

Serves 12

Preheat oven to 350°F

Crust

1 cup graham cracker crumbs

3 Tbsp sugar

1/2 tsp cinnamon

1/4 cup melted unsalted butter

Combine and press into a 9-inch spring form pan.

Cake

2 (8 oz) packages cream cheese

1/2 cup sugar

2 eggs

1/2 tsp vanilla

***

4 cups thinly sliced peeled apples

1/3 cup sugar

1/2 tsp cinnamon

1/4 cup chopped pecans

Combine cream cheese and sugar and mix at medium speed until well blended. Add eggs one at a time, mixing well. Blend in vanilla and pour over crust.

Toss apples with combined sugar and cinnamon and spoon over cream cheese layer. Sprinkle with pecans. Bake approximately 70 minutes. Loosen edges and remove rim of pan. Chill.

Thanksgiving Cheesecake

Nutrition Facts

Serving Size: (0.0g)
Servings Per Container: 12

Amount Per Serving

Calories 270   Calories from Fat 180

	% Daily Value*
Total Fat 20g	**31%**
Saturated Fat 10g	**50%**
Trans Fat 0g	
Cholesterol 80mg	**27%**
Sodium 180mg	**8%**
Total Carbohydrate 19g	**6%**
Dietary Fiber 0g	**0%**
Sugars 13g	
Protein 4g	

Vitamin A 10%	•	Vitamin C 0%
Calcium 4%	•	Iron 2%

* Percent Daily Values are based on a 2,000 calorie diet. Your daily values may be higher or lower depending on your calorie needs:

	Calories:	2,000	2,500
Total Fat	Less than	65g	80g
Sat Fat	Less than	20g	25g
Cholesterol	Less than	300mg	300mg
Sodium	Less than	2,400mg	2,400mg
Total Carbohydrate		300g	375g
Dietary Fiber		25g	30g

INGREDIENTS: CREAM CHEESE (MILK, CHEESE CULTURES, SALT, GUAR GUM), APPLES, GRAHAM CRACKERS (UNBLEACHED ENRICHED FLOUR (WHEAT FLOUR, NIACIN, REDUCED IRON, THIAMINE MONONITRATE {VITAMIN B1}, RIBOFLAVIN {VITAMIN B2}, FOLIC ACID), GRAHAM FLOUR (WHOLE GRAIN WHEAT FLOUR), SUGAR, SOYBEAN OIL, HONEY, LEAVENING (BAKING SODA AND/OR CALCIUM PHOSPHATE), SALT, SOY LECITHIN, ARTIFICIAL FLAVOR), SUGAR, EGG, BUTTER (CREAM, NATURAL FLAVOR), PECANS, CINNAMON, VANILLA EXTRACT (WATER, ALCOHOL (35%), SUGAR, VANILLA BEAN EXTRACTIVES)

Creamy Chocolate Dessert

Serves 12

1 envelope unflavoured gelatin

4 large eggs

2 cups milk

1/4 cup sugar

6 oz package semi-sweet chocolate squares, chopped

2 (1 oz) squares unsweetened chocolate, chopped

1 tsp vanilla

2 cups whipping cream

In a saucepan, beat egg yolks, milk and sugar with a whisk until blended. Sprinkle gelatin over mixture and let stand 1 minute. Stir in chopped chocolate.

Cook over low heat, stirring constantly for approximately 15 minutes until gelatin is dissolved, chocolate is melted and mixture thickens and coats a spoon. Do not boil or it will curdle.

Remove from heat. Stir in vanilla. Beat with whisk or beater until blended completely. Cover and refrigerate for 1 1/2 hours, stirring occasionally.

In a small bowl, beat whipping cream until stiff peaks form. Fold into chocolate mixture and pour into dessert dishes or ramekins. Refrigerate 4 hours or until set.

Creamy Chocolate Dessert

Nutrition Facts

Serving Size: (102g)
Servings Per Container: 12

Amount Per Serving

Calories 240   Calories from Fat 150

	% Daily Value*
Total Fat 17g	**26%**
Saturated Fat 10g	**50%**
Trans Fat 0g	
Cholesterol 90mg	**30%**
Sodium 50mg	**2%**
Total Carbohydrate 17g	**6%**
Dietary Fiber 2g	**8%**
Sugars 14g	
Protein 5g	

Vitamin A 10%	•	Vitamin C 0%
Calcium 8%	•	Iron 20%

* Percent Daily Values are based on a 2,000 calorie diet. Your daily values may be higher or lower depending on your calorie needs:

	Calories:	2,000	2,500
Total Fat	Less than	65g	80g
Sat Fat	Less than	20g	25g
Cholesterol	Less than	300mg	300mg
Sodium	Less than	2,400mg	2,400mg
Total Carbohydrate		300g	375g
Dietary Fiber		25g	30g

INGREDIENTS: MILK (PASTEURIZED REDUCED FAT MILK, VITAMIN A PALMITATE, VITAMIN D3), HEAVY CREAM (HEAVY CREAM, SKIM MILK, CARRAGEENAN), EGG, BAKER'S SEMI SWEET CHOCOLATE SQUARES, CHOCOLATE, SUGAR, GELATIN, VANILLA EXTRACT (WATER, ALCOHOL (35%), SUGAR, VANILLA BEAN EXTRACTIVES)

Lemon Pudding Cups

Serves 6

Preheat oven to 350°F

2 large eggs, separated

2 large lemons, washed

1/4 tsp salt

3/4 cup sugar, divided

1 cup milk

3 Tbsp flour

2 Tbsp unsalted butter, melted

Grate lemons to make 1 Tbsp of peel. Squeeze juice to make 1/3 cup.

In a small bowl, beat egg whites and salt to form soft peaks. Gradually add 1/2 cup sugar, beating until dissolved and you have stiff peaks.

In a large bowl, beat egg yolks and 1/4 cup sugar until blended. Add lemon juice and peel, milk, flour and melted butter. Beat until well mixed, scraping sides as needed. Fold egg whites into egg yolk mixture and pour into greased ramekins. Place in 9 x 13 glass baking dish. Fill halfway up the side of ramekins with boiling water. Bake for 40-45 minutes. Cool in fridge and serve.

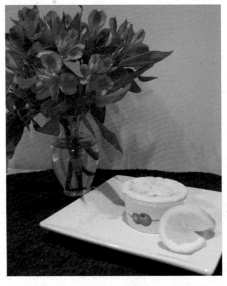

Lemon Pudding Cups

Lemon Pudding Cups

Nutrition Facts

Serving Size: (135g)
Servings Per Container: 6

Amount Per Serving

Calories 230	Calories from Fat 60

	% Daily Value*
Total Fat 6g	9%
Saturated Fat 3.5g	18%
Trans Fat 0g	
Cholesterol 75mg	25%
Sodium 140mg	6%
Total Carbohydrate 41g	14%
Dietary Fiber 2g	8%
Sugars 30g	
Protein 5g	

Vitamin A 6%	•	Vitamin C 45%
Calcium 8%	•	Iron 6%

* Percent Daily Values are based on a 2,000 calorie diet. Your daily values may be higher or lower depending on your calorie needs:

	Calories:	2,000	2,500
Total Fat	Less than	65g	80g
Sat Fat	Less than	20g	25g
Cholesterol	Less than	300mg	300mg
Sodium	Less than	2,400mg	2,400mg
Total Carbohydrate		300g	375g
Dietary Fiber		25g	30g

INGREDIENTS: MILK (PASTEURIZED REDUCED FAT MILK, VITAMIN A PALMITATE, VITAMIN D3), LEMON, SUGAR, EGG, ENRICHED UNBLEACHED FLOUR (WHEAT FLOUR, MALTED BARLEY FLOUR, NIACIN, IRON, THIAMINE, RIBOFLAVIN, FOLIC ACID), BUTTER (CREAM, NATURAL FLAVOR), SALT

Icy Dark Sweet Cherries

Serves 4

This is lovely to serve any time but especially on a hot summer day.

1 lb dark sweet cherries
6 oz semi-sweet chocolate pieces (1 cup)
1/2 cup half and half cream
3/4 tsp vanilla extract

Wash cherries, keeping stems intact. Dry and place in a single layer in a baking pan (keep them separated). Freeze. About 15 minutes before serving, remove cherries from freezer. In a saucepan, combine chocolate and cream. Cook over low heat, stirring until chocolate is melted and smooth. Remove from heat and stir in vanilla. On a plate, place chocolate in a small bowl in centre and surround with frozen cherries. Pick up by the stem and dip away.

Icy Dark Sweet Cherries

Nutrition Facts	
Serving Size: (187g)	
Servings Per Container: 4	

Amount Per Serving	
Calories 330	Calories from Fat 140

	% Daily Value*
Total Fat 15g	**23%**
Saturated Fat 9g	**45%**
Trans Fat 0g	
Cholesterol 10mg	**3%**
Sodium 20mg	**1%**
Total Carbohydrate 48g	**16%**
Dietary Fiber 5g	**20%**
Sugars 39g	
Protein 4g	

Vitamin A 4%	•		Vitamin C 15%
Calcium 6%	•		Iron 6%

* Percent Daily Values are based on a 2,000 calorie diet. Your daily values may be higher or lower depending on your calorie needs:

	Calories:	2,000	2,500
Total Fat	Less than	65g	80g
Sat Fat	Less than	20g	25g
Cholesterol	Less than	300mg	300mg
Sodium	Less than	2,400mg	2,400mg
Total Carbohydrate		300g	375g
Dietary Fiber		25g	30g

INGREDIENTS: CHERRIES, SEMI-SWEET CHOCOLATE (SUGAR, CHOCOLATE, COCOA BUTTER, MILK FAT, SOY LECITHIN, VANILLIN, ARTIFICIAL FLAVOR, MILK), HALF AND HALF (MILK, CREAM), VANILLA EXTRACT (WATER, ALCOHOL (35%), SUGAR, VANILLA BEAN EXTRACTIVES)

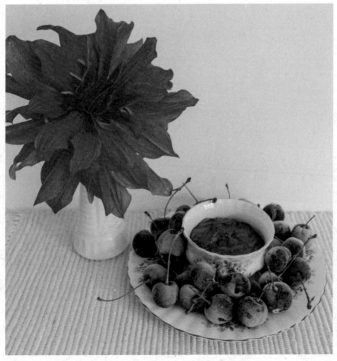

Icy Dark Sweet Cherries

Orange Chiffon Pie

Serves 8

Preheat oven to 375°F

Pie Filling

1/2 cup whipping cream

1 Tbsp icing sugar

1 tsp vanilla

1/4 cup water

1 (3 oz) package orange jello

12 oz orange-flavoured yogurt

Crust

1 1/2 cups graham cracker crumbs

6 Tbsp unsalted butter, melted

1/4 cup sugar

Mix crust ingredients in pie plate and press into bottom and sides. Bake for 8 minutes. Cool.

Pour whipping cream, icing sugar and vanilla into a large bowl. Beat until stiff peaks are formed. Set aside. Place water into a saucepan and bring to a boil. Whisk in orange jello mix until dissolved. Stir in yogurt. Fold in whipping cream. Pour into crust and refrigerate until set (1-2 hours).

Orange Chiffon Pie

Nutrition Facts

Serving Size: (107g)
Servings Per Container: 8

Amount Per Serving

Calories 300	Calories from Fat 120

	% Daily Value*
Total Fat 14g	22%
Saturated Fat 8g	40%
Trans Fat 0g	
Cholesterol 35mg	12%
Sodium 170mg	7%
Total Carbohydrate 39g	13%
Dietary Fiber 0g	0%
Sugars 27g	
Protein 6g	

Vitamin A 10%	•	Vitamin C 0%
Calcium 4%	•	Iron 2%

* Percent Daily Values are based on a 2,000 calorie diet. Your daily values may be higher or lower depending on your calorie needs:

	Calories:	2,000	2,500
Total Fat	Less than	65g	80g
Sat Fat	Less than	20g	25g
Cholesterol	Less than	300mg	300mg
Sodium	Less than	2,400mg	2,400mg
Total Carbohydrate		300g	375g
Dietary Fiber		25g	30g

INGREDIENTS: YOGURT, GREEK, STRAWBERRY, LOWFAT, GRAHAM CRACKERS (UNBLEACHED ENRICHED FLOUR (WHEAT FLOUR, NIACIN, REDUCED IRON, THIAMINE MONONITRATE {VITAMIN B1}, RIBOFLAVIN {VITAMIN B2}, FOLIC ACID), GRAHAM FLOUR (WHOLE GRAIN WHEAT FLOUR), SUGAR, SOYBEAN OIL, HONEY, LEAVENING (BAKING SODA AND/OR CALCIUM PHOSPHATE), SALT, SOY LECITHIN, ARTIFICIAL FLAVOR), JELL-O RASPBERRY GELATIN, BUTTER (CREAM, NATURAL FLAVOR), HEAVY CREAM (HEAVY CREAM, SKIM MILK, CARRAGEENAN), WATER, SUGAR, POWDERED SUGAR (SUGAR, CORNSTARCH), VANILLA EXTRACT (WATER, ALCOHOL (35%), SUGAR, VANILLA BEAN EXTRACTIVES)

Fresh Strawberry Pie

Serves 8

Preheat oven to 350°F

Crust

3/4 cup flour

3 Tbsp sugar

4 Tbsp graham cracker crumbs

1/2 cup unsalted butter

Grease pie pan. Mix together ingredients and press into bottom and sides of pie pan. Bake for 10 minutes. Cool.

Filling

1/2 quart washed, hulled and sliced strawberries

1 (6 oz) package strawberry jello

1 cup sugar

3 Tbsp corn starch

1 cup water

In a saucepan, over medium heat, cook sugar, water and corn starch until it reaches a boil. Remove from heat and stir in jello. Let cool for 10 minutes in refrigerator. Mix in strawberries and pour into pie crust. Cool in refrigerator for approximately 1 hour. Top with whipped cream if desired.

Fresh Strawberry Pie

Nutrition Facts

Serving Size: (124g)
Servings Per Container: 8

Amount Per Serving

Calories 350   Calories from Fat 100

	% Daily Value*
Total Fat 12g	18%
Saturated Fat 7g	35%
Trans Fat 0g	
Cholesterol 30mg	10%
Sodium 60mg	3%
Total Carbohydrate 60g	20%
Dietary Fiber 1g	4%
Sugars 45g	
Protein 3g	

Vitamin A 8%	•	Vitamin C 45%
Calcium 0%	•	Iron 4%

* Percent Daily Values are based on a 2,000 calorie diet. Your daily values may be higher or lower depending on your calorie needs:

		Calories:	2,000	2,500
Total Fat	Less than		65g	80g
Sat Fat	Less than		20g	25g
Cholesterol	Less than		300mg	300mg
Sodium	Less than		2,400mg	2,400mg
Total Carbohydrate			300g	375g
Dietary Fiber			25g	30g

INGREDIENTS: STRAWBERRIES, SUGAR, WATER, BUTTER (CREAM, NATURAL FLAVOR), ENRICHED UNBLEACHED FLOUR (WHEAT FLOUR, MALTED BARLEY FLOUR, NIACIN, IRON, THIAMINE, RIBOFLAVIN, FOLIC ACID), JELL-O RASPBERRY GELATIN, GRAHAM CRACKERS (UNBLEACHED ENRICHED FLOUR (WHEAT FLOUR, NIACIN, REDUCED IRON, THIAMINE MONONITRATE {VITAMIN B1}, RIBOFLAVIN {VITAMIN B2}, FOLIC ACID), GRAHAM FLOUR (WHOLE GRAIN WHEAT FLOUR), SUGAR, SOYBEAN OIL, HONEY, LEAVENING (BAKING SODA AND/OR CALCIUM PHOSPHATE), SALT, SOY LECITHIN, ARTIFICIAL FLAVOR), CORNSTARCH

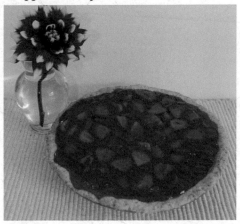

Fresh Strawberry Pie

Chocolate Cake

Serves 9

Preheat over to 350°F

Cake

1/2 cup unsalted butter

1 cup sugar

1/2 cup milk

1 tsp vanilla extract

1/4 tsp almond extract

1 cup flour

3 Tbsp corn starch

1 tsp baking powder

1/3 cup cocoa powder

4 oz egg whites (3-4 egg whites)

Grease and flour 9-inch spring form pan or 8 x 8 baking pan.

Beat butter until creamy. Add sugar and beat until light and fluffy. Add milk, vanilla and almond extract together. Sift dry ingredients together. Add milk mixture and dry mixture alternately, beating at low speed. until just blended. Set aside. Beat egg whites until stiff peaks form. Fold into cake batter and pour into prepared pan. Bake for 35-40 minutes until toothpick comes out clean. Cool. You can ice as a single layer or split in half and ice in the middle. (I like to split cake in half and spread a thin layer of icing over either side of middle sections and put a layer of raspberry preserves in between).

Chocolate Cream Icing

1/2 cup unsalted butter

1/3 cup cocoa powder

1-2 cups icing sugar (depending on consistency required)

1/4 cup half and half cream

Cream butter. Add icing sugar and cream alternately and beat until creamy. The longer you beat it the creamier it becomes (depending on the mixer 3-10 minutes). Add vanilla and beat until blended. Spread over cake.

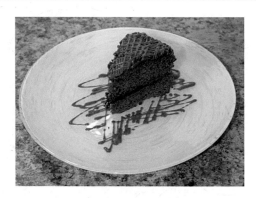

Chocolate Cake

Chocolate Cake

Nutrition Facts		
Serving Size: (85g)		
Servings Per Container: 9		
Amount Per Serving		
Calories 270	Calories from Fat 100	
		% Daily Value*
Total Fat 11g		17%
Saturated Fat 7g		35%
Trans Fat 0g		
Cholesterol 30mg		10%
Sodium 30mg		1%
Total Carbohydrate 41g		14%
Dietary Fiber 2g		8%
Sugars 26g		
Protein 4g		
Vitamin A 8%	•	Vitamin C 0%
Calcium 4%	•	Iron 6%

* Percent Daily Values are based on a 2,000 calorie diet. Your daily values may be higher or lower depending on your calorie needs:

	Calories:	2,000	2,500
Total Fat	Less than	65g	80g
Sat Fat	Less than	20g	25g
Cholesterol	Less than	300mg	300mg
Sodium	Less than	2,400mg	2,400mg
Total Carbohydrate		300g	375g
Dietary Fiber		25g	30g

INGREDIENTS: SUGAR, ENRICHED UNBLEACHED FLOUR (WHEAT FLOUR, MALTED BARLEY FLOUR, NIACIN, IRON, THIAMINE, RIBOFLAVIN, FOLIC ACID), MILK (PASTEURIZED REDUCED FAT MILK, VITAMIN A PALMITATE, VITAMIN D3), BUTTER (CREAM, NATURAL FLAVOR), EGG WHITE, COCOA, CORNSTARCH, BAKING POWDER (CORNSTARCH, SODIUM BICARBONATE, SODIUM ALUMINIUM SULFATE, MONOCALCIUM PHOSPHATE), VANILLA EXTRACT (WATER, ALCOHOL (35%), SUGAR, VANILLA BEAN EXTRACTIVES), ALMOND EXTRACT (WATER, ALCOHOL (32%), AND OIL OF BITTER ALMOND)

Chocolate Brownie Cake

This cake is more like a brownie but yummy!

Serves 12

Preheat oven to 325°F

Cake

8 eggs, yolks separated from whites
3 cups semi-sweet chocolate chips

Beat egg whites until soft peaks form. Set aside.

Grease a 9-inch spring form pan. Melt chocolate chips in a saucepan. On lowest heat, whisk in egg yolks one at a time. Remove from heat, fold in egg whites gradually. Pour into prepared pan. Put a baking sheet under in case of over flow. Bake for 30 minutes or until baked through.

Icing

1/3 cup vegetable shortening
1/3 cup cocoa powder
1 tsp vanilla
1/2 tsp almond extract
2 cups icing sugar

Beat with mixer until smooth and creamy. Spread over cake.

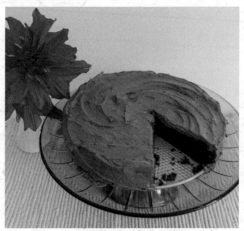

Chocolate Brownie Cake

Chocolate Brownie Cake

Nutrition Facts

Serving Size: (116g)
Servings Per Container: 12

Amount Per Serving

Calories 470   Calories from Fat 230

% Daily Value*

Total Fat 26g	**40%**
Saturated Fat 11g	**55%**
Trans Fat 0g	
Cholesterol 125mg	**42%**
Sodium 50mg	**2%**
Total Carbohydrate 55g	**18%**
Dietary Fiber 4g	**16%**
Sugars 47g	
Protein 7g	

Vitamin A 4%	•	Vitamin C 0%
Calcium 4%	•	Iron 8%

* Percent Daily Values are based on a 2,000 calorie diet. Your daily values may be higher or lower depending on your calorie needs:

	Calories:	2,000	2,500
Total Fat	Less than	65g	80g
Sat Fat	Less than	20g	25g
Cholesterol	Less than	300mg	300mg
Sodium	Less than	2,400mg	2,400mg
Total Carbohydrate		300g	375g
Dietary Fiber		25g	30g

INGREDIENTS: SEMI-SWEET CHOCOLATE (SUGAR, CHOCOLATE, COCOA BUTTER, MILK FAT, SOY LECITHIN, VANILLIN, ARTIFICIAL FLAVOR, MILK), EGG, POWDERED SUGAR (SUGAR, CORNSTARCH), OIL, VEGETABLE, NATREON CANOLA, HIGH STABILITY, NON TRANS, HIGH OLEIC (70%), COCOA, VANILLA EXTRACT (WATER, ALCOHOL (35%), SUGAR, VANILLA BEAN EXTRACTIVES), ALMOND EXTRACT (WATER, ALCOHOL (32%), AND OIL OF BITTER ALMOND)

Carrot Cake

Serves 12

Preheat oven to 350°F

Cake

2 cups all-purpose flour

1 tsp ground cinnamon

1 tsp baking powder

2/3 cup unsalted butter, softened

1 cup granulated sugar

3 large eggs

2/3 cup milk

3 medium carrots, grated

1/2 cup chopped walnuts

Icing

1/2 cup unsalted butter, softened

4 ounces cream cheese, softened

1 tsp vanilla extract

2 1/2 cups icing sugar

Grease a 9-inch round cake pan. Dust with flour. Place a baking sheet under pan to put in the oven.

Mix flour, cinnamon, baking powder together.

Beat butter and sugar together at medium speed until light and fluffy. Add eggs one at a time, beating well after each one. At low speed, alternately beat flour mixture and milk into butter mixture. Stir in carrots and nuts. Pour batter into prepared pan.

Bake until toothpick comes out clean when inserted in centre (approximately 40-50 minutes). Cool. Turn out cake onto plate.

Carrot Cake

Nutrition Facts

Serving Size: (143g)
Servings Per Container: 12

Amount Per Serving

Calories 510   Calories from Fat 250

	% Daily Value*
Total Fat 28g	**43%**
Saturated Fat 14g	**70%**
Trans Fat 0g	
Cholesterol 105mg	**35%**
Sodium 65mg	**3%**
Total Carbohydrate 60g	**20%**
Dietary Fiber 2g	**8%**
Sugars 42g	
Protein 6g	

Vitamin A 70%	•	Vitamin C 2%
Calcium 6%	•	Iron 8%

* Percent Daily Values are based on a 2,000 calorie diet. Your daily values may be higher or lower depending on your calorie needs:

	Calories:	2,000	2,500
Total Fat	Less than	65g	80g
Sat Fat	Less than	20g	25g
Cholesterol	Less than	300mg	300mg
Sodium	Less than	2,400mg	2,400mg
Total Carbohydrate		300g	375g
Dietary Fiber		25g	30g

INGREDIENTS: BUTTER (CREAM, NATURAL FLAVOR), ENRICHED UNBLEACHED FLOUR (WHEAT FLOUR, MALTED BARLEY FLOUR, NIACIN, IRON, THIAMINE, RIBOFLAVIN, FOLIC ACID), POWDERED SUGAR (SUGAR, CORNSTARCH), SUGAR, CARROTS, MILK (PASTEURIZED REDUCED FAT MILK, VITAMIN A PALMITATE, VITAMIN D3), EGG, CREAM CHEESE (MILK, CHEESE CULTURES, SALT, GUAR GUM), WALNUTS, BAKING POWDER (CORNSTARCH, SODIUM BICARBONATE, SODIUM ALUMINIUM SULFATE, MONOCALCIUM PHOSPHATE), VANILLA EXTRACT (WATER, ALCOHOL (35%), SUGAR, VANILLA BEAN EXTRACTIVES), CINNAMON

Beat butter and cream cheese at medium speed until smooth. Beat in vanilla and icing sugar until well blended.

Spread icing over cake.

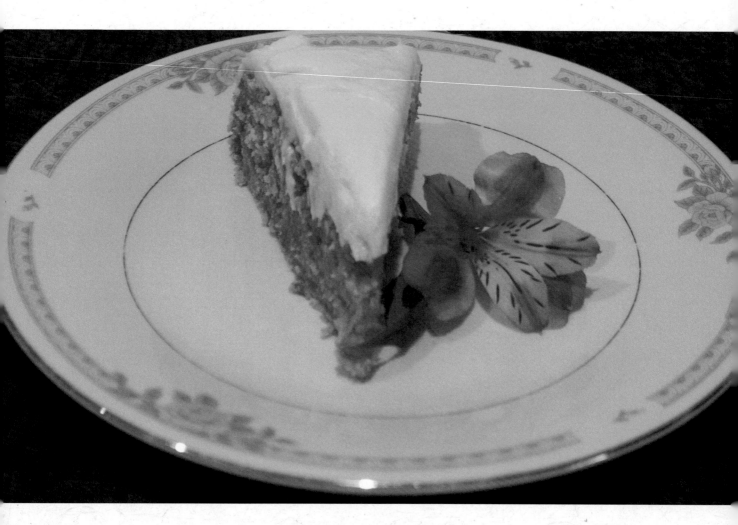

Carrot Cake

White Cake

Serves 9

Preheat oven to 350°F

1/2 cup unsalted butter

1 cup sugar

1/2 cup milk

1 tsp vanilla extract

1/4 tsp almond extract

1 1/4 cups plus 1 Tbsp flour

3 Tbsp corn starch

1 tsp baking powder

4 oz egg whites (3-4 egg whites)

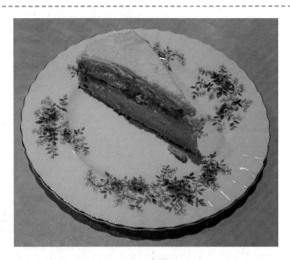

White Cake

White Cake

Grease and flour 9-inch spring form pan or 8 x 8 baking pan.

Beat butter until creamy. Add sugar and beat until light and fluffy. Add milk, vanilla and almond extract together. Sift dry ingredients together. Add milk mixture and dry mixture alternately, beating at low speed until just blended. Beat egg whites until stiff peaks form. Fold into cake batter and pour into prepared pan. Bake for 35-40 minutes until toothpick comes out clean. Cool. You can ice as a single layer or split in half and ice in the middle. (I like to split cake in half and spread a thin layer of icing over either side of middle sections and put a layer of raspberry preserves in between).

Butter Cream Icing

1/2 cup unsalted butter

3 cups icing sugar

1/8 to 1/4 cup half and half cream

1 tsp vanilla

Cream butter. Add icing sugar and cream alternately and beat until creamy. The longer you beat it, the creamier it becomes (depending on the mixer 3-10 minutes). Add vanilla and beat until blended. Spread over cake.

Nutrition Facts

Serving Size: (127g)
Servings Per Container: 9

Amount Per Serving

Calories 460   Calories from Fat 190

	% Daily Value*
Total Fat 21g	**32%**
Saturated Fat 13g	**65%**
Trans Fat 0g	
Cholesterol 55mg	**18%**
Sodium 35mg	**1%**
Total Carbohydrate 64g	**21%**
Dietary Fiber <1g	**2%**
Sugars 46g	
Protein 4g	

Vitamin A 15%	•	Vitamin C 0%
Calcium 6%	•	Iron 6%

* Percent Daily Values are based on a 2,000 calorie diet. Your daily values may be higher or lower depending on your calorie needs:

	Calories:	2,000	2,500
Total Fat	Less than	65g	80g
Sat Fat	Less than	20g	25g
Cholesterol	Less than	300mg	300mg
Sodium	Less than	2,400mg	2,400mg
Total Carbohydrate		300g	375g
Dietary Fiber		25g	30g

INGREDIENTS: POWDERED SUGAR (SUGAR, CORNSTARCH), BUTTER (CREAM, NATURAL FLAVOR), ENRICHED UNBLEACHED FLOUR (WHEAT FLOUR, MALTED BARLEY FLOUR, NIACIN, IRON, THIAMINE, RIBOFLAVIN, FOLIC ACID), MILK (PASTEURIZED REDUCED FAT MILK, VITAMIN A PALMITATE, VITAMIN D3), SUGAR, EGG WHITE, HALF AND HALF (MILK, CREAM), CORNSTARCH, VANILLA EXTRACT (WATER, ALCOHOL (35%), SUGAR, VANILLA BEAN EXTRACTIVES), BAKING POWDER (CORNSTARCH, SODIUM BICARBONATE, SODIUM ALUMINIUM SULFATE, MONOCALCIUM PHOSPHATE), ALMOND EXTRACT (WATER, ALCOHOL (32%), AND OIL OF BITTER ALMOND)

Banana Cake

- -

Serves 9

Preheat over to 350°F

1/2 cup unsalted butter

1 cup sugar

1 1/4 cups plus 1 Tbsp flour

3 Tbsp corn starch

1 tsp baking powder

4 oz egg whites (3-4 egg whites)

2 medium mashed ripe bananas

2 tsp vanilla

1/4 cup plain yogurt

3/4 cup sour milk (add lemon juice to milk)

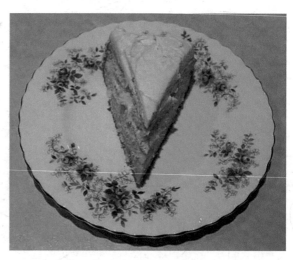

Banana Cake

Grease and flour 9-inch spring form pan

Beat butter until creamy. Add sugar and beat until light and fluffy. Sift dry ingredients together. Add milk and dry mixture alternately, beating at low speed until just blended. Add yogurt, bananas and vanilla until just blended. Beat egg whites until stiff peaks form. Fold into cake batter and pour into prepared pan. Bake for 35-40 minutes until toothpick comes out clean. Cool. You can ice as a single layer or split in half and ice in the middle.

Butter Cream Icing

1/2 cup unsalted butter

3 cups icing sugar

1/8-1/4 cup half and half cream

1 tsp vanilla

Cream butter. Add icing sugar and cream alternately, beating until creamy. The longer you beat it the creamier it becomes (depending on the mixer 3-10 minutes). Add vanilla and beat until blended. Spread over cake.

Banana Cake

Nutrition Facts

Serving Size: (181g)
Servings Per Container: 9

Amount Per Serving

Calories 550   Calories from Fat 190

	% Daily Value*
Total Fat 21g	**32%**
Saturated Fat 13g	**65%**
Trans Fat 0g	
Cholesterol 60mg	**20%**
Sodium 40mg	**2%**
Total Carbohydrate 83g	**28%**
Dietary Fiber 1g	**4%**
Sugars 63g	
Protein 5g	

Vitamin A 15%	•	Vitamin C 6%
Calcium 6%	•	Iron 6%

* Percent Daily Values are based on a 2,000 calorie diet. Your daily values may be higher or lower depending on your calorie needs:

		Calories:	2,000	2,500
Total Fat	Less than		65g	80g
Sat Fat	Less than		20g	25g
Cholesterol	Less than		300mg	300mg
Sodium	Less than		2,400mg	2,400mg
Total Carbohydrate			300g	375g
Dietary Fiber			25g	30g

INGREDIENTS: POWDERED SUGAR (SUGAR, CORNSTARCH), BANANAS, BUTTER (CREAM, NATURAL FLAVOR), SUGAR, MILK (PASTEURIZED REDUCED FAT MILK, VITAMIN A PALMITATE, VITAMIN D3), ENRICHED UNBLEACHED FLOUR (WHEAT FLOUR, MALTED BARLEY FLOUR, NIACIN, IRON, THIAMINE, RIBOFLAVIN, FOLIC ACID), EGG WHITE, HALF AND HALF (MILK, CREAM), NONFAT GREEK YOGURT (NONFAT YOGURT (CULTURED PASTEURIZED NONFAT MILK), LIVE AND ACTIVE CULTURES: S. THERMOPHILUS, L. BULGARICUS, L. ACIDOPHILUS, BIFIDUS AND L. CASEI), CORNSTARCH, LEMON JUICE, VANILLA EXTRACT (WATER, ALCOHOL (35%), SUGAR, VANILLA BEAN EXTRACTIVES), BAKING POWDER (CORNSTARCH, SODIUM BICARBONATE, SODIUM ALUMINIUM SULFATE, MONOCALCIUM PHOSPHATE)